Hairdressing: Level 1

The Interactive Textbook

An Interactive Multimedia
Blended eLearning System

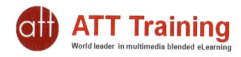

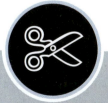

Alison Read and Charlotte Church, ATT TRAINING

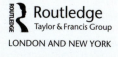

Routledge
Taylor & Francis Group

LONDON AND NEW YORK

First published 2012
by Routledge
2 Park Square, Milton Park, Abingdon, Oxon OX14 4RN

Simultaneously published in the USA and Canada
by Routledge
711 Third Avenue, New York, NY 10017

Routledge is an imprint of the Taylor & Francis Group, an informa business

© 2012 ATT Training

British Library Cataloguing in Publication Data
A catalogue record for this book is available from the British Library

Library of Congress Cataloging-in-Publication Data
Read, Alison, 1974–
Hairdressing. Level 1 : the interactive textbook / by Alison Read and Charlotte Church.
    p. cm.
Includes index.
1. Hairdressing—Textbooks. I. Church, Charlotte, 1981— II. Title.
TT972.R4178 2012
646.7′24—dc23
2012004659

ISBN: 978-0-415-52866-5 (pbk)
ISBN: 978-0-203-10694-5 (ebk)

Typeset in Helvetica
by RefineCatch Limited, Bungay, Suffolk

Contents

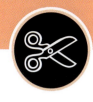

Preface

All of us at ATT Training are proud to be producing the best multimedia blended eLearning materials available for hairdressing training. We have achieved this by working with the best hairdressers, product manufacturers and salons, as well as great colleges and training centres. We started this about 15 years ago and our materials have got better every year since!

To keep improving, as well as continuing to develop our computer-based and online learning materials we are very pleased to have teamed up with a leading publisher to produce this full-colour and interactive textbook. It can be used on its own, or in conjunction with our multimedia materials online. All the essential materials are free for students and even more is available to teachers for a very low annual fee. Please contact us for details at info@atthairdressing.com

This book is the first in the 'Hairdressing: Multimedia Blended eLearning' series:

- Hairdressing – Level 1
- Hairdressing – Level 2
- Hairdressing – Level 3

As you are probably just starting out on your hairdressing career, we hope you find the content useful and informative. Comments, suggestions and feedback are always welcome at our website: www.atthairdressing.com. You will also find links to lots of free online resources to help with your studies.

We also have interesting and useful materials and ideas on these sites, come and join in:

 Facebook: www.facebook.com/atthairdressing

 Twitter: www.twitter.com/atthairdressing

 YouTube: www.youtube.com/atthairdressing

 Flickr: www.flickr.com/atthairdressing

Acknowledgements

ATT Training is grateful to the following companies and individuals for supplying assistance and/or materials and working to help with the production of our books and computer-based materials:

- Kennadys, Ingatestone, Essex (Salon of the Year winner) www.kennadys.co.uk
- Splinters, London www.splintersacademy.com
- Inter Training Service (ITS)
- Bexley College
- The Manchester College
- Wella
- L'Oréal
- Sandra Brock (consultant)
- John Cornell (photographer)
- Beth Denton
- Danielle Nott
- Freya Bennett
- Phoebe Wilkinson
- Ben Griffiths
- Sarah Reading

Pronunciation of useful words

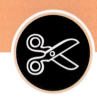

There are quite a few unusual words and phrases that we come across as hairdressers. In this short section we have listed as many as we can think of – please let us know via the website if you find any more.

To keep it simple we have not used complicated and unusual characters so our method is not perfect, but it is very close. The word is shown followed by the same word spelt phonetically (fon-et-ik-a-lee). A quick tip is that a single vowel like -o- is sounded as in 'lock' or if it is shown as -oh- then it is said as in 'broke' and if shown as -oo- then it is sounded as in 'food'.

If you have access to all our online multimedia screens then you can listen to how our narrator says the words – he gets most of them right!

Abrasion	(a-bray-shon)
Acetic acid	(a-see-tick asid)
Adhesion	(a-de-shon)
Alcohol	(al-coh-hol)
Alkaline	(al-ca-line)
Alopecia areata	(al-oh-pee-sha a-ree-ah-ta)
Alpha keratin	(al-fa keh-ra-tin)
Amino acid	(a-me-no asid)
Ammonia	(am-oh-nee-a)
Androgenic alopecia	(an-droh-jen-ik al-oh-pee-sha)
Asymmetric	(ay-sim-et-rik)
Barbicide	(bar-be-side)
Canities	(can-it-eez)
Capillary	(cap-ill-ah-ree)
Catagen	(cat-a-jen)
Ceramic	(sir-am-ic)
Cetrimide	(set-rim-ide)
Cicatrical alopecia	(sik-at-rik-al al-oh-pee-sha
Collodion	(coll-odd-ee-on)
Contraindication	(con-tra-in-dik-ay-shon)
Cysteine	(siss-teen)
Cystine	(siss-tyn)
Defamatory	(de-fam-a-tor-ee)
Dermal papilla	(der-mal pa-pil-a)
Dermatitis	(der-ma-ty-tiss)
Diffuse alopecia	(dy-fuze al-oh-pee-sha)
Di-sulphide	(dy-sull-fide)
Effleurage	(eff-lu-rage)

Epidermis	(ep-ee-der-miss)
Eumelanin	(you-mel-a-nin)
Follicle	(fol-ik-al)
Folliculitis	(fol-ik-you-ly-tiss)
Fragilitas crinium	(fraj-ill-i-tus krin-e-um)
Hexachlorophene	(hex-a-klor-oh-feen)
Hydrogen	(hy-dro-jen)
Hydrophilic	(hy-dro-fill-ik)
Hydrophobic	(hy-droh-foe-bik)
Hygroscopic	(hy-grow-skop-ik)
Keloid	(key-loyd)
Keratin	(ke-ra-tin)
Lanolin	(lan-o-lin)
Lanugo	(lan-oo-go)
Libellous	(ly-bell-uss)
Magnesium	(mag-nee-zee-um)
Medulla	(me-dull-a)
Melanin	(mel-a-nin)
Melanocytes	(mel-a-no-sites)
Monilethrix	(mon-i-lee-thriks)
Oxymelanin	(ox-ee-mel-a-nin)
Pediculosis capitis	(ped-ik-u-loh-sis cap-it-iss)
Petrissage	(pet-re-sarge)
Pheomelanin	(fee-oh-mel-a-nin)
Pityriasis capitis	(pit-ih-ry-ah-sis cap-it-iss)
Polythene	(pol-ih-theen)
Porosity	(por-ross-it-ee)
Psoriasis	(sor-rye-a-sis)
Scabies	(scay-bees)
Sebaceous cyst	(seb-ay-shus sist)
Seborrhoea	(seb-or-ee-ah)
Sodium hydroxide	(soh-dee-um hy-drok-side)
Sulphur	(sul-fur)
Telogen	(tel-oh-jen)
Tinea capitis	(tin-ee-a cap-it-iss)
Trichologist	(try-kol-oh-jist)
Trichorrhexis nodosa	(tri-kor-rex-iss noh-doh-sa)
Vellus	(vel-uss)
Zinc pyrithione	(zink py-rith-ee-on)

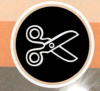

CHAPTER 1

Introduction

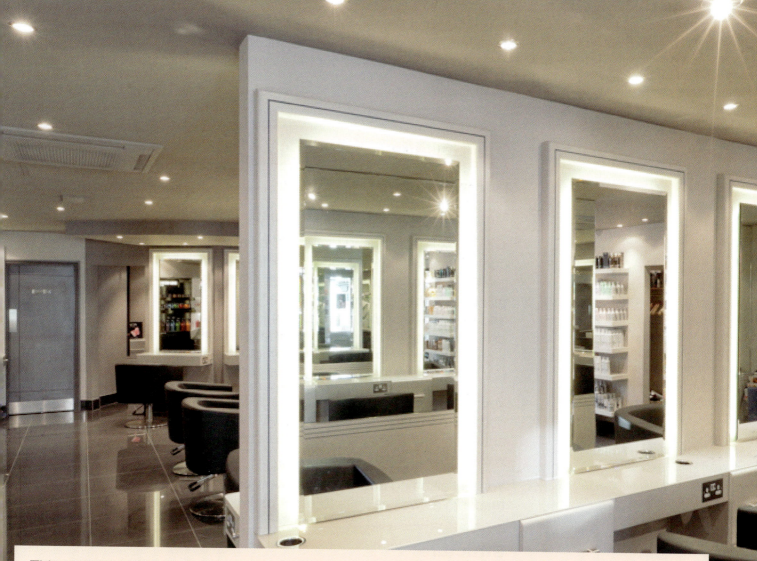

This chapter explains how to use this book. It is also a general introduction to the hairdressing industry

In this chapter you will learn about:

■ how to use this book to help you learn more and have fun in the process

■ development routes and career prospects

■ how to gain information that will help you in the industry.

Why do you want to be a hairdresser?

Well, I am sure we all have different answers to this question but I bet most are similar. My answer would have been something like: 'Because it is an amazing industry to work in. It is wide-ranging as well as being creative and you get to meet lots of really nice people.'

Hairdressing is so much more than clipping hair with scissors! Each chapter of this book therefore covers an important area such as colouring, perming, styling and more. We didn't quite get the 'Assist with shaving' unit complete in time for publication (sorry!) but the amazing multimedia screens are available online, as is a printable version of the unit.

In this first chapter we look at the information you will need to know if you wish to work as a hairdresser or barber, including career prospects, opportunities for development and gaining helpful information.

1.1 How to use this book

Introduction

Most of all, relax, take your time, and enjoy it!

This book is fine if used just on its own. However, if used in conjunction with the associated online learning material, it is even better. Most of the text and images are the same on screen and in this book – the resources on screen may be larger and animations and videos are often used. Lots of learning activities are included, either in boxes to the side, or at the end of each chapter. These are a great way to learn so complete them as you work through the book.

You may be accessing the computer-based materials through a college or training centre. However, the learning screens, questions, activities (and more!) are also available if you are at home from: www.atthairdressing.com

You will also find a forum where you can talk to other students and teachers as well as links to other useful sites and resources.

Structure

This textbook is set out in chapters that cover the mandatory and optional units needed for a qualification. Each chapter is split into sections and has activity sheets at the end. Remember, the structure of the computer-based material is exactly the same. At the start of each chapter you will find a page showing the contents with the free online multimedia materials colour coded as follows:

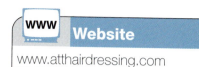

CHAPTER 2 HEALTH AND SAFETY: CONTENTS, SCREENS AND ACTIVITIES

Photographs and diagrams

Some of the photographs and diagrams in this book may need information to be added (labels, sketches, notes, etc.). Use the online or computer-based material to find out what should be added to the book. In some cases there may be a blank space where a diagram or information from the computer screen should be drawn or written.

Use this book as a workbook, make notes, underline things, make sketches and highlight important points. However, you should only do this if you own it; if it is a library or college book, use a separate piece of paper!

Margin boxes

Throughout the book you will find lots of boxes in the margins similar to the ones shown here:

Safety first

Important health and safety points will be highlighted here

Definition

Unusual words and phrases are put into this type of box

Key information

Special and important facts that you should remember will be added in boxes like this

Website

www.atthairdressing.com

Glossary

There is a comprehensive glossary at the back of this book. It is also available online at www.atthairdressing.com where you can search for important words and phrases and even translate them into other languages.

We have also added a guide to the pronunciation of unusual words in this format: (proh-nun-see-ay-shun), at the front of the book. This method is not perfect, but it will help!

Activities

Online activities are a very important part of the book and you should use them as you work through the text. When you see the following symbol, carry out the activity stated by going to the website and completing the interactive multimedia screen.

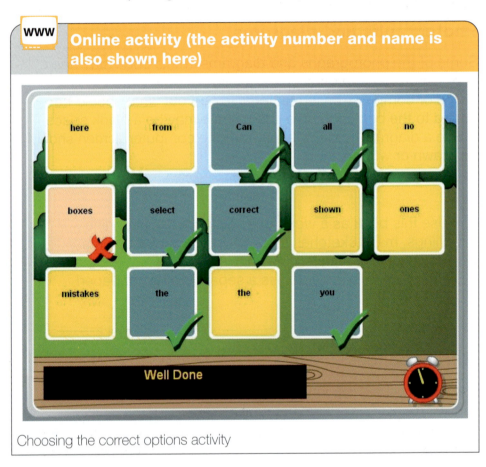

WWW **Online activity (the activity number and name is also shown here)**

here	from	Can	all	no
boxes	select	correct	shown	ones
mistakes	the	the	you	

Well Done

Choosing the correct options activity

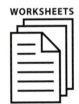
WORKSHEETS

Worksheets

As well as the 'Activity' boxes there are some paper-based worksheets at the end of each main chapter. You can carry out these tasks during your study of a chapter or unit, or at the end.

If your college or training company is registered with ATT Training, lots more activity sheets are available. Please visit www.atthairdressing.com for more details.

Assessment

There are multiple-choice quizzes available online and you should do these after you have studied a complete unit. You will see the following icon at the end of each chapter:

Online multiple-choice quiz

. . . and good luck in the final exam, which will be arranged by your tutor/assessor.

You can also print a certificate of achievement – but only if you answer all the questions correctly of course!

1.2 Development routes and career prospects

You can train to become a hairdresser or barber in the following ways:

- colleges and training providers offer full or part-time NVQ (National Vocational Qualification), SVQ (Scottish Vocational Qualification) and VRQ (Vocationally Related Qualification) courses in awards, certificates or diplomas
- trainees are taken on at salons which allow you to learn from other colleagues, take part in training in-house and attend a day-release programme at college
- if still at school then there are courses that you can become involved in which will lead you on to the above steps.

There are four different levels of work in hairdressing and therefore the training courses and qualifications are set to match these levels. This book covers the knowledge required for Level 2.

Table 1.1 Levels of work

Level 1:	Level 2:	Level 3:	Level 4:
This is often the place school leavers start and can include work such as shampooing, conditioning and helping with work such as perming and colouring as well as supporting the rest of the team and helping clients.	This can be thought of as the junior stylist or barber and will include cutting, colouring and more complex tasks.	A stylist or senior stylist will be at this level and above. It will include more complex work such as consultations as well as supervision of others.	At this level you will usually be employed in management of a large salon or arranging shows and exhibitions.

Once you are trained as a stylist you can then take short courses in specialist areas such as colouring, hair extensions etc. through manufacturers, hair shows and seminars. Some colleges and universities offer higher level qualifications once you are experienced in hairdressing. For more information you can visit the government website www.direct.gov.uk.

The salons in which we may work are many and varied, but there are also lots of other places where a good hairdresser can work. Here are some examples but I am sure there are more:

- Leisure clubs and gyms
- Health and fitness clubs
- Spa industry
- Fashion/photographic industry
- Film/television/theatre
- Clients' homes
- Cruise liners
- Clinics and hospitals
- Residential homes
- Holiday resorts and hotels
- Department stores
- Product manufacturers and suppliers
- Product house representative

The type of career path we take can also be varied. Vidal Sassoon, Nicky Clarke and Lee Stafford all started at the bottom and worked their way to the top. We won't all do that, but just being a good stylist in a salon is a great job, or you may end up running your own salon or working in television or films.

Here are some examples of more varied roles in our industry that may interest you:

- Trichologist:
  Clients with scalp or hair disorders may need to be referred to a doctor, but in many cases a trichologist, who is a specialist in hair and scalp disorders, may be the best choice. It takes a few years to qualify but can be a fascinating career.

- Management:
  Many hairdressers go on to run their own salon, which means you will need management skills. You could also take on a managerial role in a large salon or even manage training courses for new students.

- TV, Film and Theatre:
  The creative industries are difficult to get into as there are not many openings. However, never let that put you off, if you are determined you will get there in the end with enthusiasm and hard work.

- Manufacturers:
  The large manufacturers need sales representatives, technical representatives and demonstrators for their products.

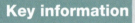

Key information

Vidal Sassoon, Nicky Clarke, Lee Stafford and many other top hairdressers all started at the bottom and worked their way up.

- Teaching:
  A career in teaching a skill such as hairdressing usually follows significant experience in the industry and will also require additional qualifications.
- Writing books and learning materials:
  And of course you may have ambitions to write a book!

Whatever career path you follow in hairdressing it will be interesting, challenging and exciting, so go on out there and have fun!

1.3 Helpful information

This section explains the services that are offered, job roles available and how you can become a hairdresser/barber. If more information is needed then some organisations that can help are highlighted throughout this section.

Gaining information about the hairdressing industry

If you are interested in training to become a hairdresser, you can find information from:

- the Internet
- magazines/trade journals
- course leaflets/prospectuses
- education and training providers
- awarding bodies such as City & Guilds, VTCT, Edexcel
- job centres
- organisations specialising in professional career guidance
- shows/seminars
- advertisements/word of mouth
- work experience
- Habia (sector skills council).

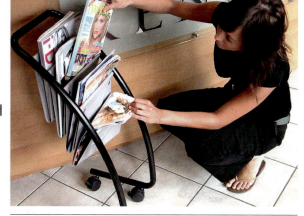

Figure 1.1 Magazines and trade journals provide valuable information

Hairdressing salons do not just offer haircutting services. They offer a great range of services. The different types of salon will offer their own types of services. They do not often offer all of the services as it is based on their clients' wishes.

Occupational roles within the hair industry

You should understand all the job titles and roles in the salon. These include:

- shampooist
- junior/trainee
- receptionist
- junior stylist/stylist
- colour technician

Key information

Hairdressing services may include:

- shampooing and conditioning
- cutting and blow drying
- styling and dressing
- colouring
- perming
- relaxing
- shaving
- facial haircutting
- face massage
- scalp massage
- Indian head massage.

- artistic director
- manager
- salon owner
- barber.

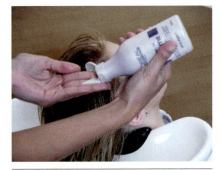

Figure 1.2 Dispensing shampoo

Shampooist

The shampooist, as the name suggests, shampoos the client's hair and prepares them for the stylist. They may also look after the washbasin area.

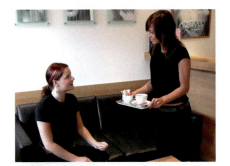

Figure 1.3 A junior/trainee will assist clients by getting refreshments for example

Junior/trainee

The junior or trainee works under the direction of a higher ranking member of staff. They help with many different tasks including assisting with clients (getting refreshments, taking coats etc.), shampooing, perming, colouring, styling, blow drying and reception duties.

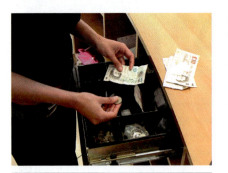

Figure 1.4 The receptionist will take payment

Receptionist

The receptionist attends to visitors and enquiries, answers the telephone, takes bookings for appointments, takes and records payments for services and retail items. He/she will also maintain the reception area.

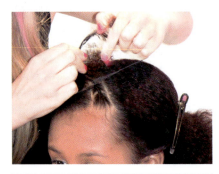

Figure 1.5 The stylist provides hair care services to enhance appearance

Junior stylist/stylist

The junior stylist will carry out only basic hairdressing services on the client, guided by a stylist. The stylist provides hair care services to enhance the client's appearance. They deliver a wide range of services including giving advice, styling, cutting and colouring.

Colour (chemical) technician

The colour technician specialises in the application of tint to clients' hair. Therefore they have an in-depth knowledge of the use of chemicals in salons. Many will also offer other chemical services, for example perming and relaxing.

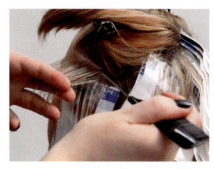

Figure 1.6 The colour technician specialises in the application of colour

Artistic director

Artistic directors are responsible for all hairdressing design work. This will include any publicity and promotional work for the salon. They also help with management of the salon and training of staff.

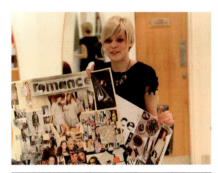

Figure 1.7 Artistic directors are responsible for design work

Manager

The manager participates in the smooth running of the salon on a day-to-day basis. He/she is normally responsible for:

- overseeing the team in the salon
- employing staff
- organising training and promotions
- ordering supplies
- paying bills.

It is up to the salon manager to ensure the salon is a profitable business whilst adhering to health and safety legislation.

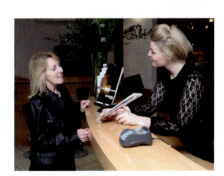

Figure 1.8 The manager ensures that the salon runs smoothly

Salon owner

The salon owner may also be the manager of the salon and he/she usually carries out a wide range of business tasks. Many salon owners will also style clients' hair.

Tasks that the owner may carry out include:

- hiring employees
- dealing with customer queries/complaints
- overseeing health and safety policy and legal requirements
- ordering stock and supplies
- pricing retail products
- making new business
- managing finances.

Figure 1.9 The salon owner will deal with customer enquiries

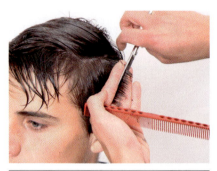

Figure 1.10 Barbers specialise in men's hair

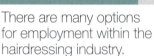
Key information

There are many options for employment within the hairdressing industry.

Barber

Barbers specialise in the styling of men's hair. This includes cutting hair and maintaining facial hair or shaving.

Employment characteristics

There are many different options when working in the hair industry. Your employment characteristics could be as follows:

- full or part-time
- self-employed
- employed seasonally.

Some staff are only employed on certain days of the week, for example on a Saturday. This may be the case early on in your career. Your hours of work can vary from day to day. Many salons have 'late night openings' on certain days and you may be required to work until closing. Renting a chair is another choice that you may be given at some point through your hairdressing career. This allows you to be self-employed and you would pay the salon to use their space and facilities.

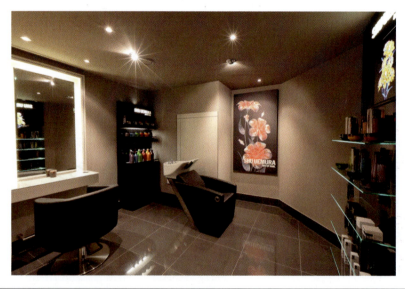

Figure 1.11 You may rent a chair within a salon

Career patterns

Your first role when you start working in the hairdressing industry will usually be as a trainee. From here you can progress to becoming a stylist, then a senior stylist. Once you have reached this stage you can then move into management if you wish. The speed of your progression will not only depend on the training and qualifications you achieve but also how well you work within the salon. Most salons have their own career progression paths that you will follow once you start working.

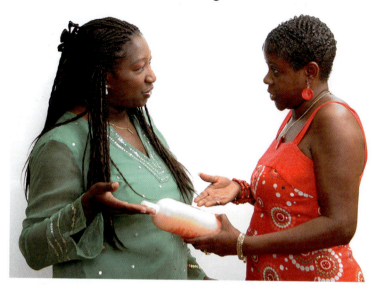

Figure 1.12 You will usually start work as a trainee

Organisation types

As a hairdresser you may need to access the following organisations:

- salons
- professional membership organisations
- industry lead bodies
- manufacturers and suppliers.

Salons

Salons offer hairdressing services and products to meet clients' requirements. A great deal of experience can be gained working in a salon whilst training to become a hairdresser or barber.

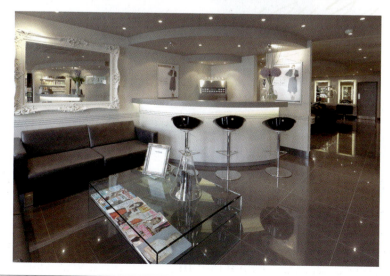

Figure 1.13 A salon (Kennadys in Ingatestone, Essex)

Professional membership organisations

One of the roles of this type of organisation is to allow hairdressers or barbers to be state registered. Becoming a SRH (state registered hairdresser) gives you official recognition under the Hairdressers Registration Act. The Hairdressing Council is an example of this type of organisation. Professional membership organisations will also provide information about ethical issues and legislation within the industry.

Industry lead bodies

The main role of the lead body organisations (or sector skills councils) is to set the standards for a particular industry (i.e. hair and beauty). Qualifications are formed from these standards. These bodies are appointed by the government.

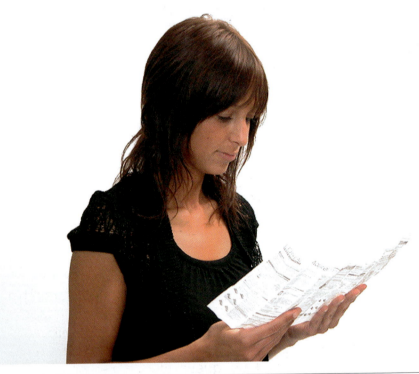

Figure 1.14 Lead bodies set standards which form qualifications

Manufacturers and suppliers

These organisations make and supply products and other equipment (i.e. brushes, hair dryers, rollers etc.) that salons both use and sell on to the client. You may come into contact with manufacturers and suppliers if you have to return items, check their pricing or find out the ingredients of products.

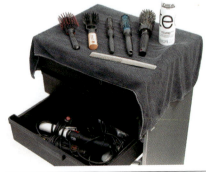

Figure 1.15 Manufacturers make the products used in the salon

1.4 Preparing for assessments

1.4.1 Simple steps

Assessment can be stressful time for a student. However, there are some simple steps you can take to increase your confidence and performance:

1. Study the course materials as you are going along – don't leave it all to the last minute!
2. Nearer to the exam/assessment, set aside a certain time each day to practise and study
3. Take advantage of all pre-test material in this book, online and of course any that your teacher provides
4. Attend all revision sessions even if you feel you don't really need it
5. Ask your teacher to clear up any uncertainties
6. Take time off work a few days before your assessment to allow extra time to study
7. Sleep well the night before the assessment/exam
8. Eat a healthy breakfast the morning of your assessment to help you wake up and get your brain working
9. Don't put too much pressure on yourself to perform
10. Don't 'cram' too much at the last minute (for you will almost certainly forget things if you do)
11. Remember, if you worked hard to get this far you can only do your best.

1.4.2 Multiple-choice tests

Multiple-choice exams are easy for some and hard for others. The best thing about a multiple-choice quiz is that all the information you will need is given to you. The downside is that the additional information given to you is designed to make sure you really know the correct answer – and don't just guess. Here are some tips on how to prepare for a multiple-choice test:

- Practise, practise, practise
- Do the online quizzes and other examples of the tests several times to get used to the format
- Read all the answer options, it is often possible to rule out one or two easily so that then even if you need to guess, you have a 50:50 chance of getting it right!
- Answer ALL the questions – don't miss any out.

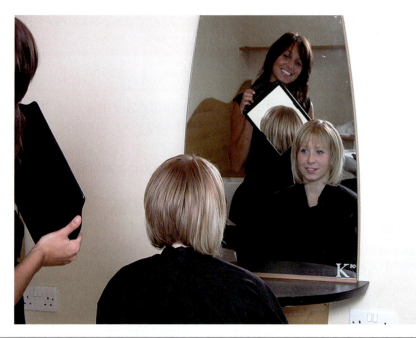

Figure 1.16 On reflection, you will do fine in your exams . . .

1.4.3 Practical exams

Practical work is clearly the most important part of being a hairdresser. For this reason you will have to do a number of practical examinations or tests either in your college or at your salon. These are often described as observed assessments.

If you only read one part of this section make sure it is this bit:

For your practical assessments you should:
- have a professional attitude
- look the part – be smart, clean and looking good
- not have doubts about your abilities; it will show – so be confident
- not allow other students to influence you, concentrate on your work not on that of others
- pause, relax and take a moment if you forget a procedure or process – it will come back to you
- relax and don't panic!

Remember, the job of your assessor or examiner is to make a professional judgement that you have met the necessary standards and are therefore competent to do your job. They do not want to fail you, but of course they will ensure you have reached the necessary standard before saying you have passed. It is easy to feel intimidated because the assessor will not talk much and will be making notes. This is not designed to put you off, it is to make sure they are fair to everyone and that they judge you against set criteria.

They may ask you some oral questions during or after the assessment procedure. Don't panic, take your time and answer clearly and confidently.

- If you have practised and studied hard during your training – the assessments will be easy – I promise!

Personal appearance

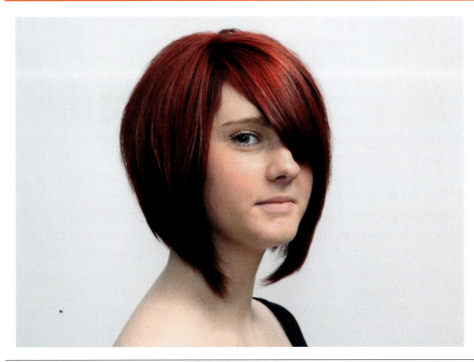

Figure 1.17 Look good, feel good

Now, there is an old saying that I am sure you agree with: *'If you look good you feel good'.* In addition, your appearance should show the 'client' (model and an assessor in this case) that you are capable of caring for your own appearance, therefore are capable of caring for others.

Here are some important tips; you may like to add notes after each one such as how you will prepare yourself and what you will wear:

- **Shoes** – your footwear should be comfortable, clean, polished if appropriate and in good repair (so no trainers and flip-flops then!)
- **Clothes** – these should be professional in appearance, clean, ironed and comfortable (so no jeans and jogging suits then!)
- **Hair** – it is very important that your own hair looks good and it should be clean and styled. Showing your assessor/examiner/ client that you look after your own appearance is important (so no bed-heads then!)
- **Facial hair** – men should ensure that they are either clean shaven or that your beard or moustache is neatly shaped and trimmed (so no one-day stubble then!)
- **Make-up** – don't overdo it, make sure it is practical and appropriate for a day's work. Maybe just a soft shade of lipstick

and some light mascara would be ideal? (Guys using make-up is fine, but don't overdo it either!)

- **Fresh breath** – if necessary use breath mints, but don't chew gum; it is very unprofessional (so, you may need to get that appointment at the dentist too!)
- **Perfume or cologne or aftershave** – in a salon, either at your work or at college, there will be many other people and odours from different products. Some clients may be allergic or sensitive to strong scents (so, the floral perfume from gran is probably not the best choice!)
- **Nails** – you should avoid extreme nails as they can be distracting. They should be practical so that you can carry out the procedures required for your assessments. Nails should be clean and cared for (so don't bite them during the exams!)
- **Personal hygiene** – no client, model or examiner wants to be close to a hairdresser with bad body odour. Bath or shower daily, use deodorant and change clothes regularly (so don't jog five miles on your way to the exam!)
- **Jewellery** – keep this to a minimum, too many rings and bracelets will prevent you working properly. Excessive body jewellery such as facial piercings can be distracting (but, don't refuse that diamond engagement ring!)
- **Mobile phones** – these should always be turned off when working; in fact for an exam they may be prohibited (so, not on vibrate, turn it off!)

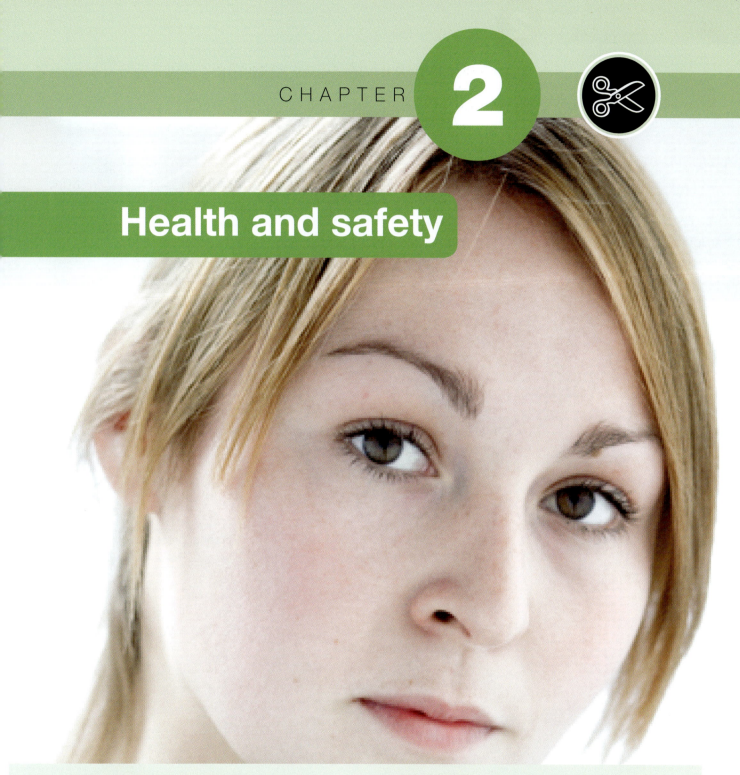

Health and safety

This chapter covers the NVQ/SVQ unit G20, Make sure your own actions reduce the risk to health and safety; and VRQ unit 202, Follow health and safety in the salon

In this chapter you will learn about supporting health and safety in the workplace. Health and safety is the responsibility of all persons at work. Employers and supervisors in particular have a greater responsibility for health and safety than trainees. Staff should be aware of their own competence levels in the workplace. All staff should not only adhere to legal responsibilities but also manufacturers' and workplace instructions whilst keeping in mind environmental issues at all times.

In this chapter you will learn about:

- identifying the hazards and evaluating the risks in your workplace

- reducing the risks to health and safety in your workplace.

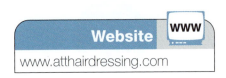

CHAPTER 2 HEALTH AND SAFETY: CONTENTS, SCREENS AND ACTIVITIES

Key:
Sections from the book are set in this colour
Screens available online are set in this colour
Online activity screens are set in this colour

Hazards and risks at work

Introduction
Likely hazards
Risks associated with the hazards and avoiding

Identify the risks
Displaying rules and regulations
Five in a row

Reduce risks to health and safety at work

Introduction
Health and Safety at Work Act 1974 (1)
Health and Safety at Work Act 1974 (2)
Select Correct Bars
COSHH 1
COSHH 2
Precautions
Manual Handling Operations Regulations 1992
Lifting 1
Lifting 2
Electricity at Work Regulations 1989
RIDDOR 1996
Dermatitis
The Provision and Use of Work Equipment Regulations 1998
Personal Protective Equipment at Work Regulations 1992
Workplace Regulations 1992
Operate safely in the salon 1
Select correct boxes
Operate safely in the salon 2
Equipment
Methods of sterilisation
Disposal of waste
First aid
Round the board
First aid problems
Fire
Fire safety

General rules
Emergency fire procedure
Fire extinguishers
Correct selection
Calling emergency services
Periodic checks
Other emergencies
Security
Recording accidents
Select correct group
Client care
Client records
Data protection
Personal presentation and hygiene 1
Personal Presentation and hygiene 2
Five in a row
Jewellery
Posture and deportment
Exercise and rest
Worksheet – First aid
Worksheet – Personal protective equipment (PPE) at work regulations
Worksheet – Dermatitis
Worksheet – Hazards and risks
Worksheet – Legislation
Worksheet – Control of substances Hazardous to Health (COSHH) Regulations
Worksheet – sterilisation
Online multiple choice quiz

2.1 Hazards and risks at work

Likely hazards

Many things around the salon can be a hazard. A hazard is a source of danger. Examples of hazards include:

- electrical equipment
- storage boxes
- products
- trailing leads.

Hazards should be identified, acted upon and reported depending on the individual salon policy. This is to minimise the risk of accidents. You should know the right person to approach if there is a health and safety problem or a risk of one.

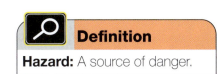

Definition

Hazard: A source of danger.

Risks associated with the hazards and avoiding these risks

The risk is the likelihood of an accident occurring from a hazard.

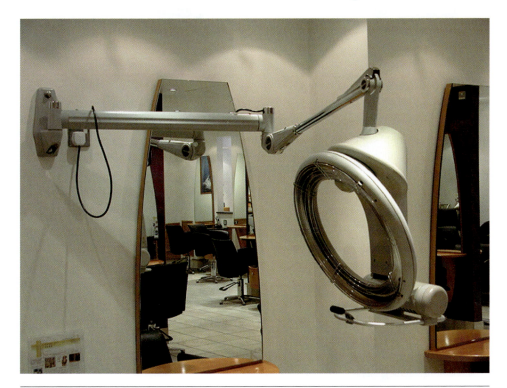

Figure 2.1 Electrical equipment

One risk from electrical equipment is that it will cause somebody an injury when using or repairing it. To avoid this happening it is important that staff are trained in its use and the equipment is tested to make sure it is in the correct working order.

Storage boxes may be a risk if they are stored in front of a fire exit for example. There is a strong likelihood that they will cause an accident. The boxes must be moved to an area that does not cause a risk to injury.

Products may cause a risk if they contain chemicals that are flammable and toxic. They must be stored securely and only be available to hairdressers who have been trained in their use.

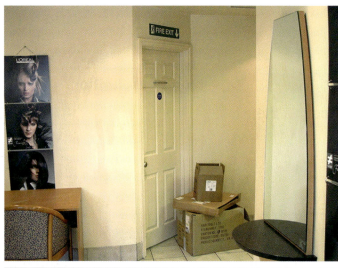

Figure 2.2 Storage boxes

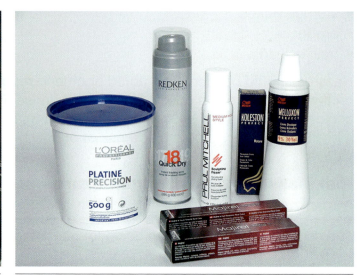

Figure 2.3 Products

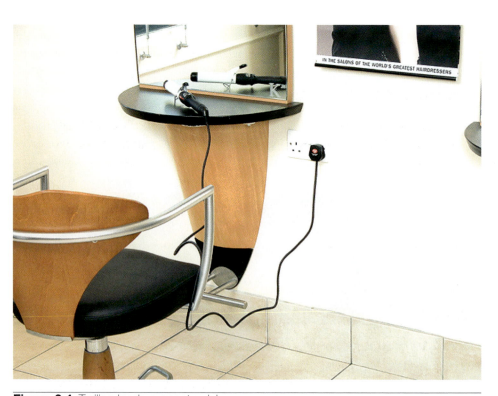

Figure 2.4 Trailing leads present a risk

Key information

The risk is the likelihood of an accident occurring from a hazard.

Trailing leads are a risk if it is likely that somebody may trip over them. Make sure they are not in the way of a client or another member of staff.

Identify the risks

You must be able to identify risks and understand the actions that should be taken to avoid an accident occurring (risk assessment).

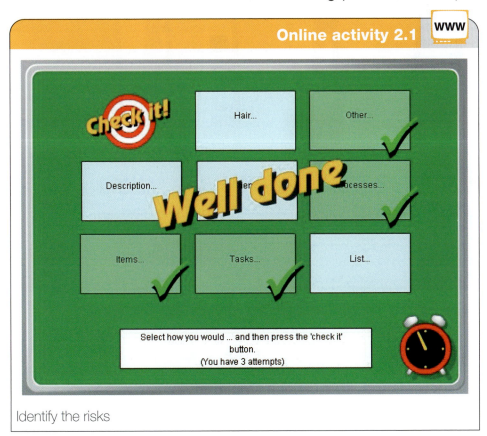

Identify the risks

Displaying rules and regulations

Every salon must, by law, display the rules and regulations of its health and safety on the wall in a position that can be seen by everyone.

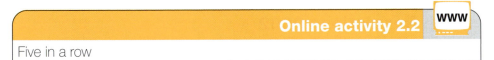

Five in a row

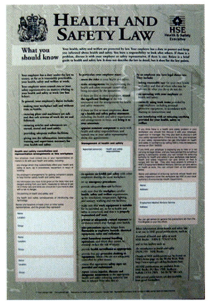

Figure 2.5 Rules and regulations poster

2.2 Reducing risks to health and safety at work

In order to reduce the risks to health and safety in your workplace, certain legislation must be followed. It is also important to act in accordance with the health and safety policies that the salon operates, manufacturers'/suppliers' instructions and also your own competence levels. Doing this at all times will significantly reduce the risks, thus allowing you to control them.

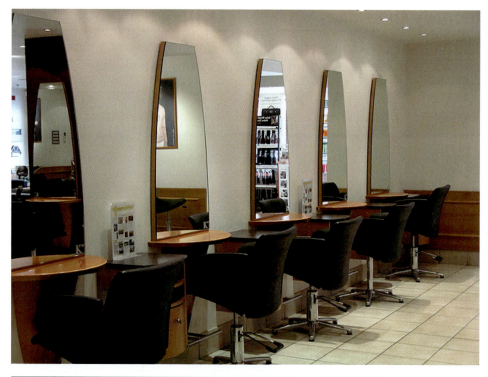

Figure 2.6 Act accordingly with health and safety policies in the salon

The Health and Safety at Work Act 1974

This Act places a strict duty on employers to ensure, so far as is reasonably practicable, safe working conditions and the absence of risks to health in connection with the use, handling, storage and transport of articles and substances.

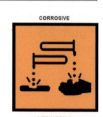

WWW **Online activity 2.3**

Correct selection

Control of Substances Hazardous to Health Regulations 2002

These are commonly called the COSHH regulations and they lay down the essential requirements for controlling exposure to hazardous substances and for protecting people who may be affected by them.

A substance is considered to be hazardous if it can cause harm to the body. It only poses a risk if it is:

- inhaled (breathed in)
- ingested (swallowed)
- in contact with the skin
- absorbed through the skin
- injected into the body
- introduced into the body via cuts etc.

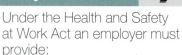

Key information

Under the Health and Safety at Work Act an employer must provide:

- safe equipment and safe systems of work
- safe handling, storage and transport of substances
- a safe place of work with safe access and exit
- a safe working environment with adequate welfare facilities
- all necessary information, instruction, training and supervision
- all necessary personal protective equipment free of charge.

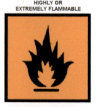

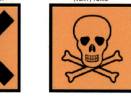

HIGHLY OR EXTREMELY FLAMMABLE   CORROSIVE

HARMFUL / IRRITANT   (VERY) TOXIC

Figure 2.7 Hazardous substance symbols showing that materials are flammable, corrosive, harmful/irritant and (very) toxic

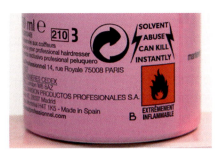

Figure 2.8 Hazardous symbol shown on a product

Precautions

- Follow manufacturers' instructions.
- Always wear personal protective equipment.
- Avoid contact of the chemical with skin, eyes and face.
- Do not use on sensitive or damaged skin.
- Always use a non-metallic bowl to avoid rapid decomposition of the product.
- Store the product in a cool, dry place away from sunlight or other sources of heat, make sure containers are properly sealed when not in use.
- Store the product in the container and replace the cap immediately after use.
- Never mix products unless recommended by the manufacturer.
- Rotate stock.
- Keep products, especially aerosols, away from naked flames or heat.

Key information

Under the COSHH regulations employers must:

- identify substances in the workplace which are potentially hazardous
- assess the risk to health from exposure to the hazardous substances and record the results
- make an assessment as to which members of staff are at risk
- look for alternative less hazardous substances and substitute if possible
- decide what precautions are required
- introduce effective measures to prevent or control the exposure
- inform, instruct and train all members of staff
- review the assessment on a regular basis.

 Website

www.atthairdressing.com

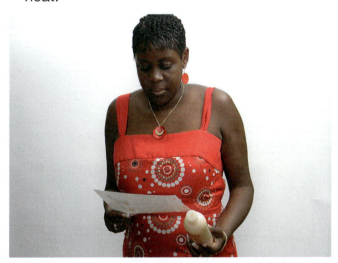

Figure 2.9 Always read manufacturers' instructions

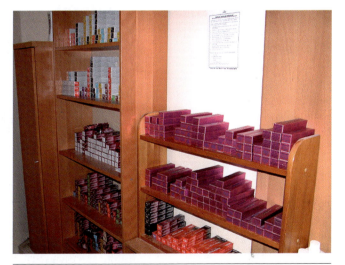

Figure 2.10 Store products in a cool, dry place away from sunlight

Manual Handling Operations Regulations 1992

These regulations cover the lifting of loads as well as lowering, pushing, pulling, carrying and moving them, whether by hand or other bodily force. You should carry out an assessment of the risks involved by looking at the following:

2

Safety first

When lifting heavy packages keep your back straight, feet slightly apart and bend your knees.

- the weight of the load
- the shape of the load (e.g. some loads may not be particularly heavy but can be awkward to lift)
- the working environment (e.g. if the area is damp the employee's hands could be wet and the load might slip)
- where the task is to be carried out (e.g. are there cramped conditions which make it difficult to lift)
- the individual's capability.

If packages are too heavy, politely ask another member of staff to help you.

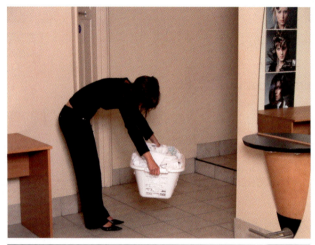

Figure 2.11 Incorrect lifting

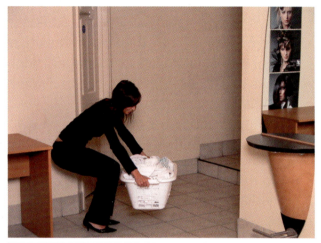

Figure 2.12 Correct lifting

Lifting

If you send a member of staff to collect stock or equipment, for example from a wholesaler or another salon, make sure that:

- the member of staff has suitable car insurance
- the member of staff is capable of lifting the stock or equipment without difficulty.

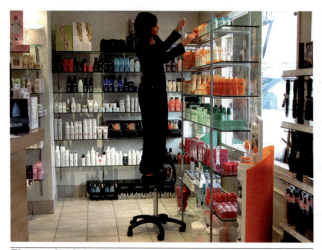

Figure 2.13 Incorrect method of lifting from a shelf

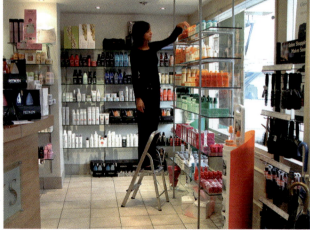

Figure 2.14 Correct method of lifting from a shelf

Electricity at Work Regulations 1989

These regulations state that you must:

- always check electrical equipment before using. Look for loose wires and make sure that the plug is not cracked or damaged in any way. Check that the cord is not frayed or cracked
- never use electrical equipment with wet hands
- electrical equipment should be maintained regularly and checked by a suitably qualified person. Once checked, the equipment should have a certificate or label acknowledging it
- faulty electrical equipment in the workplace must be removed, labelled as faulty and reported to the relevant person.

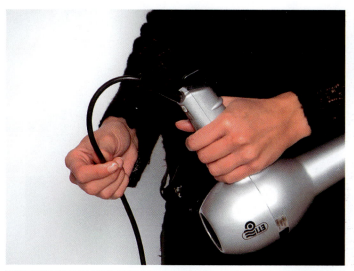

Figure 2.15 Checking electrical equipment for damage

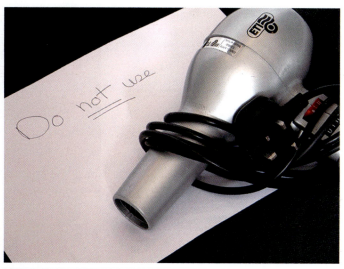

Figure 2.16 Correct labelling of faulty equipment

Reporting of Injuries, Diseases and Dangerous Occurrences Regulations Act 1996 (RIDDOR)

The Act states that work-related accidents, diseases and dangerous occurrences must be reported. You must keep these records for three years and they can be in written form and kept in a file, or a computer file.

Dermatitis

This is a very common skin disease in hairdressers and is caused by hands being exposed to certain products and carrying out wet-work regularly. Dermatitis can be prevented by:

- ensuring shampoo and conditioner are rinsed from your hands
- drying hands thoroughly
- moisturising regularly
- wearing disposable gloves.

Key information

RIDDOR records must include:

- date and method of reporting
- date, time and place of event
- personal details of those involved
- a brief description.

Safety first

Dermatitis is a reportable disease.

Definition

Dermatitis: Inflammation of the skin resulting from irritation from an external agent.

The Provision and Use of Work Equipment Regulations 1998

The following requirements apply to all equipment:

- work equipment must be suitable for the purpose for which it is used
- equipment must be properly maintained and a maintenance log kept, for example for portable electrical hand tools
- users and supervisors of equipment must be given adequate health and safety training and written instructions where required.

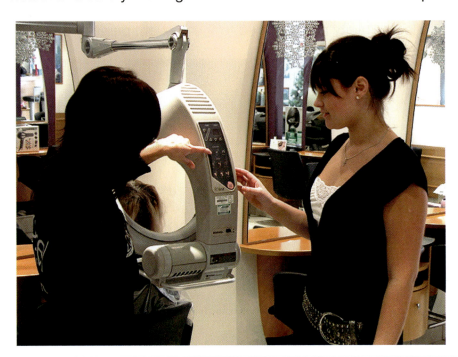

Figure 2.17 Users of equipment must be given adequate health and safety training

Personal Protective Equipment at Work Regulations 1992 (PPE)

The requirements under this Act will be met when you comply with the COSHH regulations. These regulations require every employer to provide suitable personal protective equipment (PPE) to each of his or her employees who may be exposed to any risk while at work.

The PPE supplied must be properly maintained and the users must be trained and monitored to ensure that the PPE is properly used. Employees are required to report to the employer any loss of, or damage to, PPE.

In the average salon, PPE will involve the use of gloves and wearing tinting aprons when handling perm lotion, relaxers, tints and bleach, and possibly eye protection when handling and mixing strong bleach solutions. It is the duty of the workforce to use PPE when required.

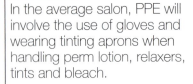

Key information

In the average salon, PPE will involve the use of gloves and wearing tinting aprons when handling perm lotion, relaxers, tints and bleach.

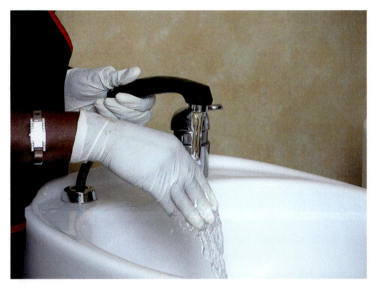

Figure 2.18 PPE equipment

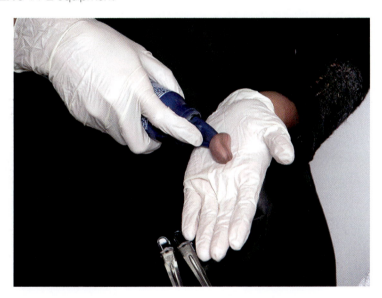

Figure 2.19 Gloves and aprons should be worn when handling chemicals

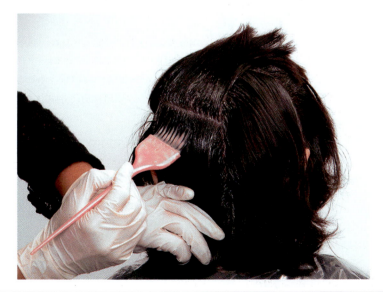

Figure 2.20 Gloves must be worn when colouring hair

The Workplace (Health Safety and Welfare) Regulations 1992

This Act states that the employer is to provide a safe working environment for employees and members of the public. The employer must legally:

- maintain equipment
- regulate temperature
- ensure adequate lighting.

Operate safely in the salon

Micro-organisms cannot be seen but are found in air, clothing, and dirt, on the surface of the skin and under the nails. Some of them can cause disease and are said to be infectious. Micro-organisms need warmth, moisture and food to multiply; all of these are present in salon conditions, so it is very important to keep the working environment clean.

They are divided into three groups:

- fungi
- bacteria
- viruses.

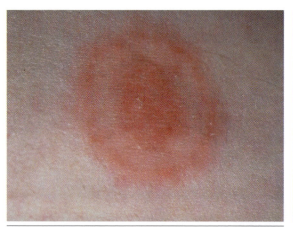

Figure 2.21 Ringworm is from the fungi group

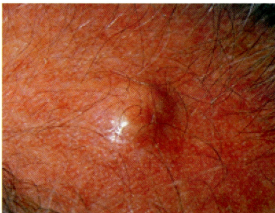

Figure 2.22 Boils are from the bacteria group

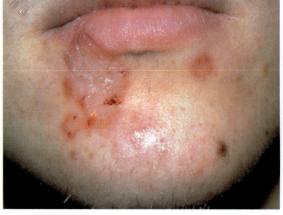

Figure 2.23 Impetigo is from the bacteria group

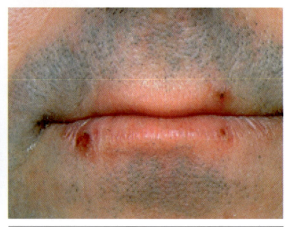

Figure 2.24 Cold sores are from the virus group

Make sure the working environment is clean and dry at all times; this includes clothing, work areas and all equipment. Floors should be kept clean; hair clippings should be swept up to prevent disease and accidents. If floors are wet, notices should be left to warn clients and other staff. Surfaces should be washed down once a day. Mirrors should be cleaned before the clients arrive.

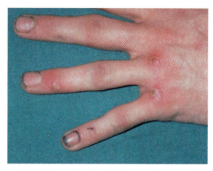

Figure 2.25 Warts are from the virus group

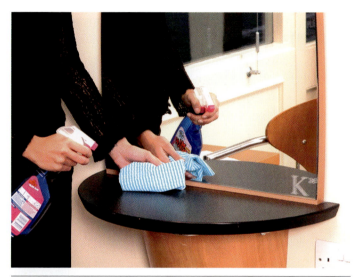

Figure 2.26 Clean work surfaces and mirrors

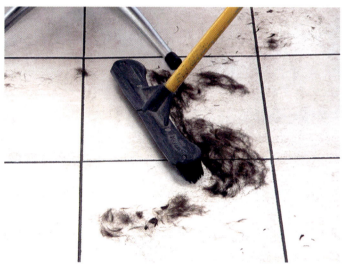

Figure 2.27 Sweep up hair clippings

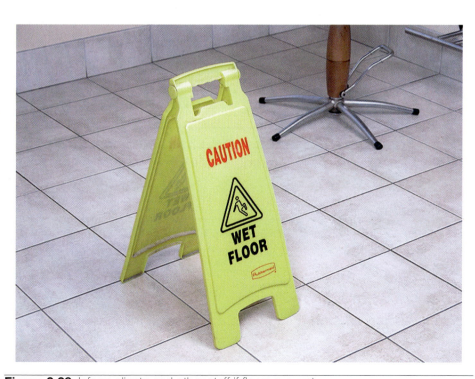

Figure 2.28 Inform clients and other staff if floors are wet

2

Definitions

Ringworm: A highly contagious fungal skin infection.

Lice: Tiny insects that are spread by head-to-head contact.

Impetigo: Contagious bacterial skin disease.

Equipment

Always use fresh, clean and sterile towels and gowns for each client. All towels should be washed after each client. Keep the used towels in a closed container. This prevents cross-infection of fungal diseases such as ringworm of the head (tinea capitis) or infestations of lice (pediculosis capitis). Bacterial diseases are also spread from dirty towels, especially impetigo.

Brushes and combs should be washed after use. All other equipment should have hair clippings removed and be cleaned carefully.

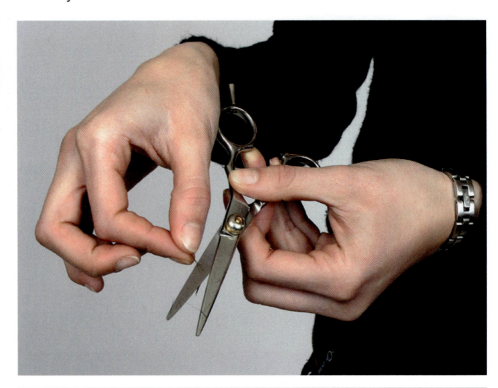

Figure 2.29 Remove hairs from scissors after use

Key information

Remember to always wash brushes and combs before sterilising.

Methods of sterilisation

Salons may use a variety of ways to sterilise equipment (make free of micro-organisms). Remember to always wash brushes and combs before sterilising.

Autoclave (heat)

This is the recommended method of sterilisation for small metal items. The high temperature steam produced destroys all micro-organisms.

UV cabinet (ultraviolet radiation)

Clean tools can be stored in a UV cabinet once they have been sterilised.

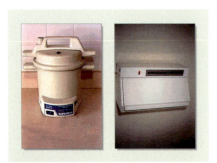

Figure 2.30 Autoclave and UV cabinet

Chemical sterilisation

Proprietary sterilising solutions and sprays are available for sterilising equipment. To be effective the chemical solutions should be used for the correct length of time and mixed using the manufacturers' instructions. Sterilising sprays are used for wiping scissors and clippers.

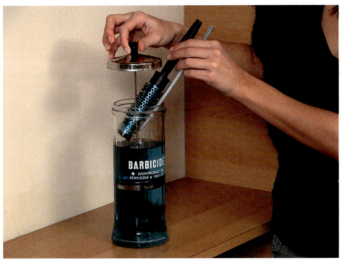

Figure 2.31 Chemical sterilising solution

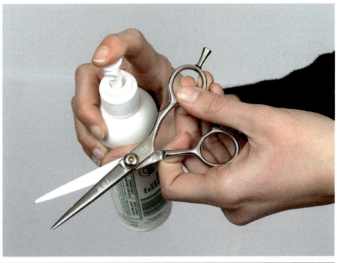

Figure 2.32 Sterilising spray

Disposal of waste

Salons produce waste as do other businesses. This waste will have a negative effect on the environment and can cause pollution. In order to reduce this, it should be managed correctly.

Covered waste bins which contain a polythene bin liner should be used for everyday items of salon waste. These should be emptied daily or when full.

Razor blades and any other sharp items should be kept away from general salon waste and placed in a safe closed container before disposal.

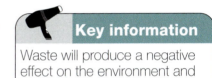

Key information

Waste will produce a negative effect on the environment and can cause pollution.

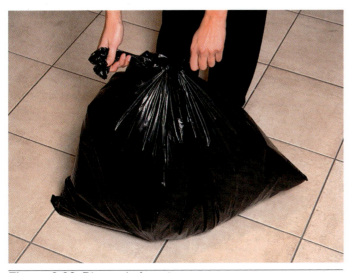

Figure 2.33 Disposal of waste

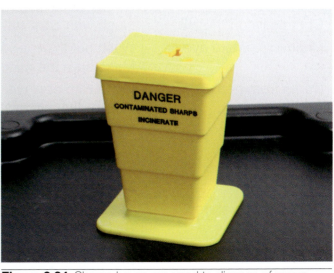

Figure 2.34 Sharps boxes are used to dispose of razors

Definition

RIDDOR: Reporting of Injuries, Diseases and Dangerous Occurrences Regulations Act.

Key information

Ensure that you are wearing gloves when performing basic first aid and you ONLY carry out basic first aid.

First aid – Regulations for First Aid 1981

All establishments should have a registered first-aider. Ensure you know the registered first-aider in your salon and where the first aid box is kept. The health and safety regulations RIDDOR require the salon to have a first aid kit available. The box is green with a white cross on it.

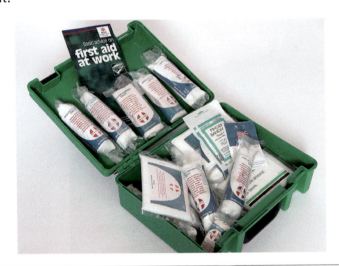

Figure 2.35 First aid box

WWW Online activity 2.5

Round the board

First aid problems

If an accident occurs in the salon, you should have a basic knowledge of what to do. The table below shows some common first aid problems and the action to take if they occur.

Table 2.1 Problems and actions

Problem	Action taken
Chemicals on the skin	Flush with cool water
Chemical enters eye	Wash out the eye with cool water until first-aider arrives Make sure the water is clean
Burns from heat	Flush with cool water Call for first aid assistance if needed
Burns from chemicals	Remove any clothing that is contaminated as long as it is not stuck to the skin Flush with cool water Call for first aid assistance if needed
Unconscious state	Put into recovery position Call for first aid assistance
Cut to the skin	Put pressure on the area using pad from first aid box If a deep cut or bleeding does not stop, call for first aid assistance

Fire

Accidents involving fire are very serious. If a fire should break out the priority is to remove clients to safety. If it is a small fire it can be extinguished with a glass fibre 'fire' blanket or an extinguisher. If the fire is too big or clearly out of control: GET OUT – STAY OUT – CALL THE FIRE BRIGADE OUT!

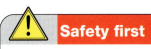

Safety first

If a fire should break out the priority is to remove clients to safety.

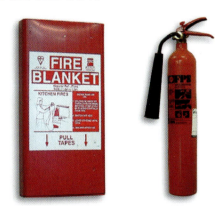

Figure 2.36 Fire blanket and fire extinguisher

Fire safety

🔍 **Definition**

Flammable: Can catch fire.

Fire precautions that should be carried out include:

- checking that exits are not obstructed
- doors to escape routes are not closed
- fire doors are kept closed but not locked
- fire fighting equipment is available and in working order
- the correct type of fire extinguisher is readily available.

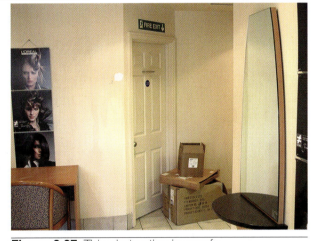

Figure 2.37 This obstruction is unsafe

General rules

The following rules can help to prevent fires:

- a 'no smoking' policy inside salons should be supported
- towels should not be placed over heaters
- electrical sockets should not be overloaded
- electrical wires should not be bare or frayed
- switch off electrical appliances when not in use
- store flammable liquids away from heat
- do not obstruct electric or gas heaters.

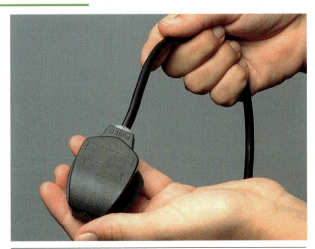

Figure 2.38 Check electrical wires

Emergency fire procedure

If a fire does happen your workplace should have a set procedure so, for example, you should know:

- How is the alarm raised?
- What does the alarm sound like?
- What do you when you hear the alarm?
- What is your escape route from the building?
- Where do you go to assemble?
- Who is responsible for calling the fire brigade?

Fire extinguishers

These can be dangerous if used incorrectly or on the wrong type of fire. They are colour coded to allow easy recognition. The table below shows the substances each type contains and the uses.

Black and blue extinguishers are recommended for the salon because they are suitable for use with electrical equipment and flammable liquids.

Safety first

Ensure that you know the emergency fire procedures in your workplace.

Safety first

All extinguishers have instructions written on them, read them now before it is too late.

Table 2.2 Fire extinguisher colours and use

Colour label	Substance	Use
Red	Water	Wood, paper, textiles, not electrical
Black	CO_2	Flammable liquids, safe for all voltages
Green	Vaporising liquids	Flammable liquids, safe for all voltages
Blue	Dry powder	Flammable liquids, safe for all voltages
Cream	Foam	Flammable liquids, not electrical

www   Online activity 2.6

Correct selection

Calling emergency services

If it is necessary to call out the emergency services then follow these rules:

- do not panic
- dial 999
- speak slowly and clearly
- tell the operator which service or services you require
- give your name, address and telephone number
- give relevant details of the fire, accident etc.
- listen and answer questions carefully
- if the fire brigade has been requested, wait in a safe place for their arrival.

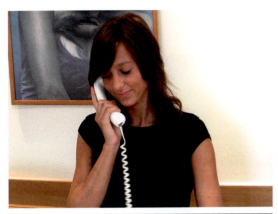

Figure 2.39 Speak slowly and clearly when calling for help!

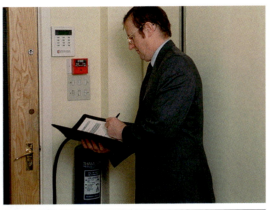

Figure 2.40 Your salon should have periodic checks by the fire prevention officer

The salon owner or employer should authorise periodic checks by the fire prevention officer. The fire brigade will offer help and advice on fire safety, evacuation procedures and choice of fire fighting equipment.

Other emergencies

Study this table to see what action you should take in certain situations.

Table 2.3 Emergencies and actions

Emergency	Action
Flood	• Turn off water • Alert the fire brigade Make sure you know where the mains stopcock is.
Bomb alert	• Phone emergency services • Evacuate
Gas leak	• Open windows • Phone emergency services • Evacuate
Suspicious person and/or package	• Report to the manager

Security

Employees should:
- lock doors at night
- close and secure windows at night
- keep the back door closed during salon hours
- never leave money or valuables unattended or in the salon overnight
- look out for unauthorised or suspicious people in the salon
- not leave the till open and unattended
- make sure clients' handbags, jewellery etc. remain with them at all times

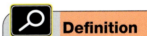

Definition

Periodic: Occurring at intervals.

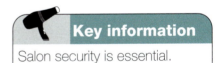

Definition

Stopcock: A valve that opens and closes a gas or water supply pipe.

Key information

Salon security is essential.

- mark their own equipment
- always report to your manager if in any doubt.

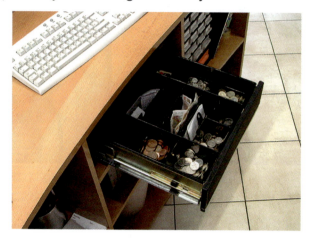

Figure 2.41 Don't leave tills open like this!

Recording accidents

All salons should have an accident book. All accidents should be recorded in the accident book.

www   **Online activity 2.7**

Drag into correct group

Client care

The client should be cared for throughout their time at the salon. Remember to:

- gown the client properly to protect their clothing
- remove all obstacles when clients are moving around the salon to prevent accidents
- make sure the client's handbag, jewellery etc. are kept with the client at all times
- take care when using products which are hazardous
- if the client needs to be evacuated whilst in the middle of a treatment always cover their hair with a towel.

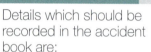
Key information

Details which should be recorded in the accident book are:

- full name and address of casualty
- date and time of the accident
- accident details
- signature of the person making the entry.

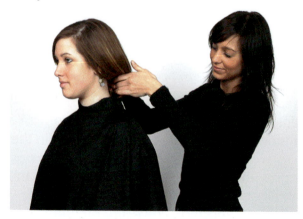

Figure 2.42 Gowning the client

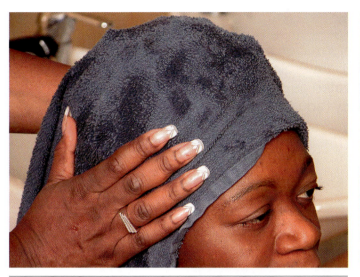

Figure 2.43 Covering client's head with a towel

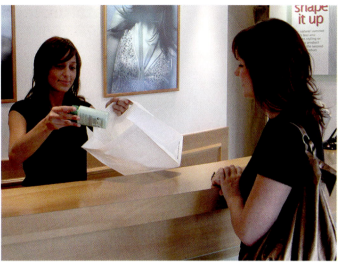

Figure 2.44 Make sure clients carry their possessions at all times

Client records

Client records should be updated regularly with all relevant details, for example if a client has had an allergic reaction to a chemical used in the salon. This can prevent an accident occurring at a later date. Record home care products sold to the client with date of purchase.

 Safety first

Client records should be updated regularly with all relevant details, for example if a client has had an allergic reaction to a chemical used in the salon.

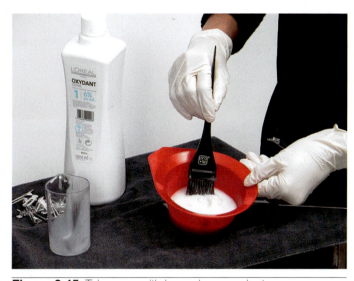

Figure 2.45 Take care with hazardous products

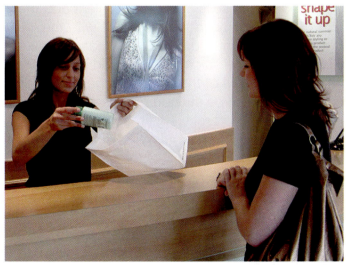

Figure 2.46 Make sure you record if a client has bought any products

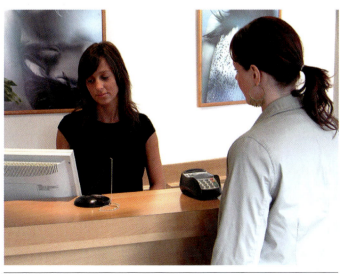

Figure 2.47 Update client records

Key information

Clients must have access to their details if they request it.

Definition

Data Protection Act: An Act that grants rights for individuals regarding the obtaining, use, holding and disclosure of information about themselves.

Data protection

If you keep client information on a computer, the company must be registered with the Data Protection Register. The information must be accurate and treated as confidential. Clients must have access to their details if they request it.

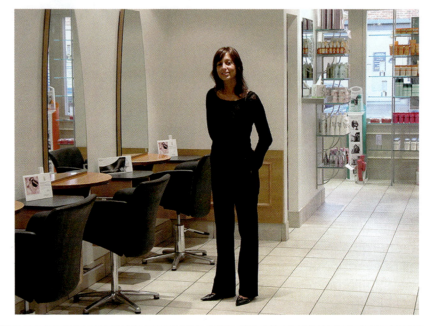

Figure 2.48 Ensure your personal hygiene and presentation is of a high standard

Personal presentation and hygiene

A stylist must always ensure his or her own personal hygiene and presentation is of a high standard. This includes:

- Hair – your hair and makeup should reflect the standards of the salon. It should be clean, fashionable and smart.
- Clothing – salon dress should reflect the style of the salon; however, it should also protect the hairdresser, be comfortable and clean. Clothing that is too loose is a risk to the client and the stylist. There is a risk of clothing coming into contact with the client or being caught in equipment. Some salons wear overalls as they lend an air of efficiency to the salon. They should protect the clothing, match the colour scheme of the salon and be neat, clean and attractive. Clothes should not be stained or creased. When colouring, perming, neutralising and relaxing an apron should be worn for extra protection. Always wash your salon clothes/overalls when they are dirty or smelly, do not wait until the end of the week.
- Mouth and teeth – bad breath is unpleasant to clients. Regular visits to the dentist will guard against bad breath. Certain foods will make your breath smell; don't eat pickled onions at lunchtime. Brush your teeth regularly. If you smoke, try to give it up.
- Hands and nails – both should be clean as the risk of spreading infection is then minimised. They should not be stained with hair colourant. Nails should not be bitten and should not be too long

(dirt can get trapped underneath). Wear disposable gloves where necessary.

- Shoes – should be comfortable and allow feet to breathe. Leather shoes would be ideal. Cut down on foot odour by washing tights or socks frequently. Hair in the salon can harm the skin. It may break the surface of the skin leaving the hairdresser open to risk of infection. The wearing of open toed shoes will increase the risk of infection.

- The skin – a bath or shower every day is essential because of the hot, humid atmosphere of the salon and the close contact the hairdresser has with the client. Always use deodorant or an antiperspirant (reduces underarm sweating). A little perfume is pleasant but too much can be overpowering.

Online activity 2.8
Five in a row

Jewellery

This should at no time interfere with the client's comfort, only the minimum of jewellery should be worn. Jewellery may scratch client's skin. It may also react with the chemicals, possibly contributing to the development of contact dermatitis.

Posture and deportment

The back should be kept straight, bend from the knees, feet apart with weight evenly distributed. If the spine is bent the back will have excess strain and the body will tire. The lungs will also be constricted; this lowers the intake of oxygen, which induces tiredness. Poor posture looks sloppy and will not give a good impression of the hairdresser.

 Safety first

Jewellery may react with chemicals, possibly contributing to the development of contact dermatitis.

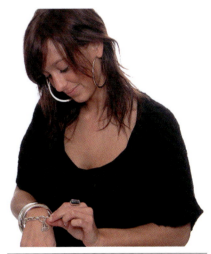

Figure 2.49 This is too much jewellery

 Safety first

The back should be kept straight, bend from the knees, feet apart with weight evenly distributed.

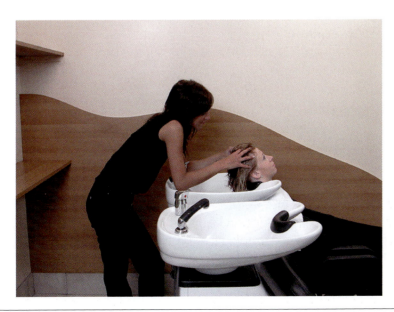

Figure 2.50 Incorrect posture

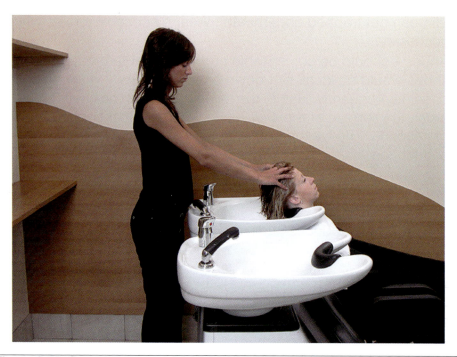

Figure 2.51 Correct posture

Exercise and rest

Hairdressing means standing for long hours so it is necessary to be fit and healthy. Exercise is vital to health; it firms muscles and moves joints keeping the body supple. During sleep, the body regenerates its energies refreshing the brain and the body. Lack of sleep reduces the quality of life when awake.

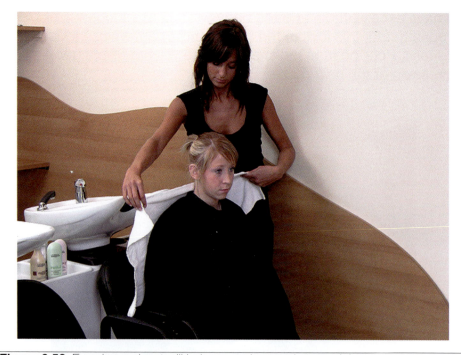

Figure 2.52 Exercise and rest will help you to be good at your job

Now complete all the worksheets in the following section.

2.3 Worksheets

You can carry out these worksheets during your study of a chapter or unit, or at the end. If your college or training company is registered with ATT Training, lots more of these worksheets are available. Write your answers directly in the book – but only if you own it of course – if it is a library or college book, use a separate piece of paper!

First aid

Regulations for First Aid 1981

All establishments should have a registered first-aider. Ensure you know the registered first-aider in your salon and where the first aid box is kept. The health and safety regulations RIDDOR require the salon to have a first aid kit available. The box is green with a white cross on it.

Who is the first-aider in your salon?

Where is the first aid kit kept in your salon?

First aid problems

If an accident occurs in the salon, you should have a basic knowledge of what to do. Ensure that you are wearing gloves when performing basic first aid and that you ONLY carry out basic first aid. When filled in, the following table will show some common first aid problems and the action to take if they occur.

Complete the following table by referring back to this chapter, or with the help of the online learning screens. Add any other information that you can think of.

Problem	Action taken

Personal protective equipment (PPE) at work regulations

The requirements under this act will have been met when you comply with the COSHH regulations.

These regulations require every employer to provide suitable personal protective equipment (PPE) to each of his or her employees who may be exposed to any risk while at work.

The PPE supplied must be properly maintained and the users must be trained and monitored to ensure that the PPE is properly used.

Employees are required to report to the employer any loss of or damage to PPE.

In the average salon, PPE will involve the use of gloves and wearing tinting aprons when handling perm lotion, relaxers, tints and bleach. Eye protection may also be necessary when handling and mixing strong bleach solutions. It is the duty of the workforce to use PPE when required.

List all of the PPE equipment you may need to use, and where you would find it in your salon, below:

Dermatitis

This is a very common skin disease in hairdressers and is caused by hands being exposed to certain products and carrying out wet-work regularly. Dermatitis can be prevented by:

- ensuring shampoo and conditioner are rinsed from your hands
- drying hands thoroughly
- moisturising regularly
- wearing disposable gloves.

Find out more about dermatitis by searching the web and make some notes below:

Hazards and risks

Hazards should be identified, acted upon and reported depending on the individual salon policy to minimise the risk of accidents.

You should know the right person to approach if there is a health and safety problem or risk of one.

Many things around the salon can be a hazard. A hazard is a source of danger.

Make a list of examples of hazards that might exist in your salon:

Legislation

You need to be aware of legislation regarding health and safety in your workplace. The legislation aims to reduce any risks that may occur. Always follow all health and safety policies operated by your salon to reduce any further risk to yourself, colleagues or clients.

Health and Safety at Work Act

This Act places a strict duty on employers to ensure, so far as is reasonably practicable, safe working conditions and the absence of risks to health in connection with the use, handling, storage and transport of articles and substances.

Under the Health and Safety at Work Act an employer must provide (add notes to each bullet):

- safe equipment and safe systems of work

- safe handling, storage and transport of substances

- a safe place of work with safe access and exit

- a safe working environment with adequate welfare facilities

- all necessary information, instruction, training and supervision

- all necessary personal protective equipment free of charge

Control of Substances Hazardous to Health (COSHH) Regulations

These are commonly called the COSHH Regulations and they lay down the essential requirements for controlling exposure to hazardous substances and for protecting people who may be affected by them.

A substance is considered to be hazardous if it can cause harm to the body. It only poses a risk if it is:

- inhaled (breathed in)
- ingested (swallowed)
- in contact with the skin
- absorbed though the body
- injected into the body
- introduced into the body via cuts etc.

Here is a picture of Mr COSHH. Label him and write about situations that may occur in your salon that could cause you to be at risk from a hazardous substance. Also make a note of actions you can take to avoid this from happening. Use the online learning screens to help you.

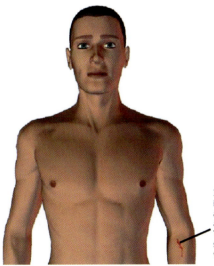

If I have an open wound it is possible that I may allow a harmful substance to be absorbed into my body. To avoid this, I should make sure any cuts are covered up with a plaster.

Figure 2.53 Mr COSHH!

Under the COSHH Regulations employers must (add notes to each bullet point):

- identify substances in the workplace which are potentially hazardous

- assess the risk to health from exposure to the hazardous substances and record the results

- make an assessment as to which members of staff are at risk

- look for alternative less hazardous substances and substitute if possible

- decide what precautions are required

- introduce effective measures to prevent or control the exposure

- inform, instruct and train all members of staff

- review the assessment on a regular basis

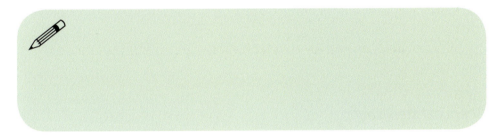

Here are some symbols to look out for:

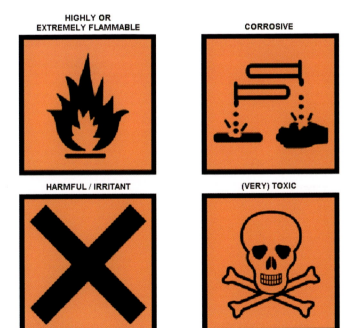

Figure 2.54 Warning symbols

Sterilisation

Salons may use a variety of ways to sterilise equipment (make free of micro-organisms). Remember to always wash brushes and combs before sterilising.

Listed below are three different types of sterilisation methods. State when each method should be used in the salon.

Autoclave (heat)

UV cabinet (ultraviolet radiation)

Chemical sterilisation

2.4 Assessment

Well done! If you have studied all the content of this unit you may be ready to test your knowledge.

Check out the 'Preparing for assessments' section in Chapter 1 if you have not already done so, and always remember:

- You can only do your best if you have . . .
  - studied hard
  - completed the activities
  - completed the worksheets
  - practised, practised, practised
  - and then revised!

Now carry out the online multiple-choice quiz

. . . and good luck in the final exam, which will be arranged by your tutor/ assessor.

Working relationships

This chapter covers the NVQ/SVQ unit G3, Contribute to the development of effective working relationships

Having good working relationships with clients and staff in the salon is paramount when working in hairdressing. This unit looks at the skills needed for creating effective relationships with clients and staff in order to improve your own personal performance.

In this chapter you will learn about:

- developing effective working relationships with clients

- developing effective working relationships with colleagues

- developing yourself within the job role.

CHAPTER 3 WORKING RELATIONSHIPS: CONTENTS, SCREENS AND ACTIVITIES

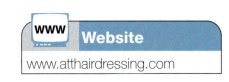

Key:

Sections from the book are set in this colour

Screens available online are set in this colour

Online activity screens are set in this colour

Develop working relationships with clients

Introduction

Develop effective relationships with clients

Communicate information to clients

Verbal communication

Non-verbal communication

Check it

Client comfort

Handling client's possessions

Referring client's concerns

Personal presentation and hygiene 1

Personal presentation and hygiene 2

Five in a row

Develop working relationships with colleagues

Introduction

Assisting others

Asking for help

Round the board

Develop yourself within your job role

Introduction

Job description

Select correct boxes

Appraisals

Self-appraisal

Strengths, weaknesses and targets

Short and long-term goals

Five in a row

Training and keeping skills up-to-date

Shadowing

Asking others for help

Setting yourself a personal training plan

Review your training plan

Select correct bars

Appeals and grievances

Worksheet – Good communication

Worksheet – Develop effective working Relationships withc

Worksheet – Setting yourself a personal training plan

Online multiple choice quiz

3.1 Develop working relationships with clients

Developing a professional attitude with clients is very important.

Communicate information to clients

Good communication in the salon is always important, especially if a business is to succeed. Communication can be in the following forms: verbal, non-verbal or written. You should be aware of your own communication and that of your clients in order to judge how they are feeling.

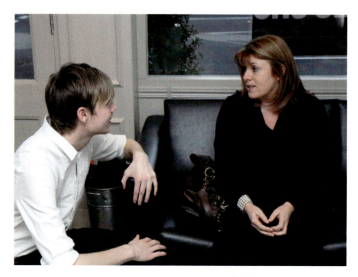

Figure 3.1 Verbal communication with a client

Verbal communication

This is spoken information. You will talk to clients and other staff members in the salon. Always speak clearly, be polite, check the information received is correct and pass to the appropriate person, if required.

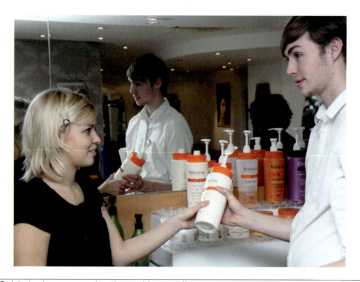

Figure 3.2 Verbal communication with a colleague

Non-verbal communication

This is the way we convey information without speaking and is also referred to as body language. Body language is a very important form of communication. Our stance, gestures or facial expressions say a lot about how we are feeling, for example smiling implies friendliness and frowning implies hostility. Maintain eye contact with the client when talking and listening to show you are paying attention and to convey friendliness and trust. Always listen carefully to the client, making sure you take in everything they are telling you.

Key information

Body language is a very important form of communication.

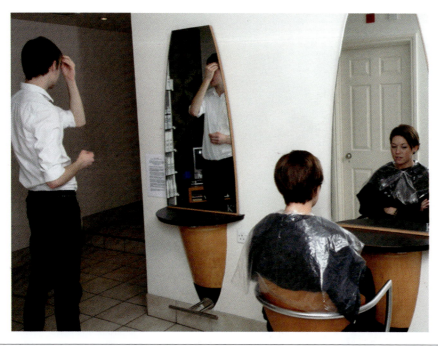

Figure 3.3 This is incorrect body language, the client is obviously upset

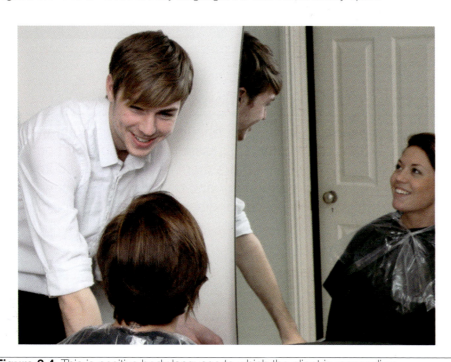

Figure 3.4 This is positive body language to which the client is responding

www **Online activity 3.1**

Check it

Client comfort

Ensure the client is comfortable and ask whether you can help with anything. This will help the client to trust you and the service you are providing. Maintain client confidentiality at all times. Do not talk about the client or give out client details such as telephone numbers.

Definition 🔍

Confidentiality: To keep secret.

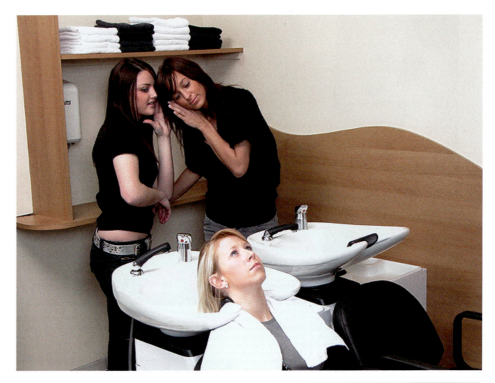

Figure 3.5 Do not gossip about clients!

Handling clients' possessions

You may be asked to help the receptionist by assisting them with clients. If handling the clients' possessions including their coats and bags, make sure that you store them carefully and securely. Bags should be placed on the floor and coats should be hung up. You should return the clients' belongings when they ask for them or at the end of the service.

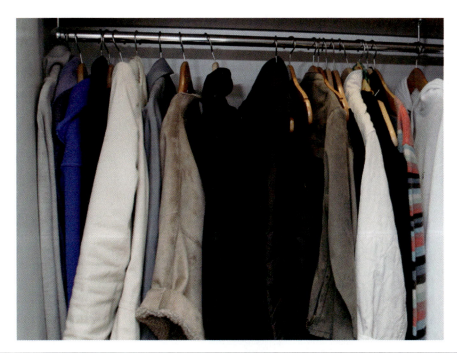

Figure 3.6 Hang coats up carefully

Referring clients' concerns

Most of the time you will be able to help the client, for example they might ask you for a drink. If you cannot help with the request (e.g. if the client asks about their colouring service) you can always ask another member of staff to help you. Never pretend to know answers to questions if you do not. It is much more professional to say you do not know the answer but you will find out from someone who does.

 Safety first

Never pretend to know answers to questions if you do not! You should say you do not know the answer but you will find out from someone who does.

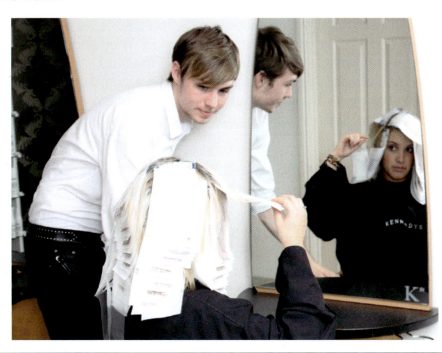

Figure 3.7 Answer questions if you can

Personal presentation and hygiene

You must always ensure your own personal hygiene and presentation is of a high standard.

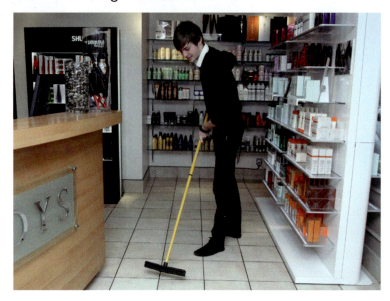

Figure 3.8 Ensure your own presentation is of a high standard at all times

This includes:

- Hair – your hair and makeup should reflect the standards of the salon. It should be clean, fashionable and smart.
- Clothing – salon dress should reflect the style of the salon; however it should also protect the hairdresser, be comfortable and clean. Clothing that is too loose is a risk to the client and the stylist. There is a risk of clothing coming into contact with the client or being caught in equipment. Some salons wear overalls as they lend an air of efficiency to the salon. They should protect the clothing, match the colour scheme of the salon and be neat, clean and attractive. Clothes should not be stained or creased. When colouring, perming, neutralising and relaxing an apron should be worn for extra protection. Always wash your salon clothes/overalls when they are dirty or smelly, do not wait until the end of the week.
- Mouth and teeth – bad breath is unpleasant to clients. Regular visits to the dentist will guard against bad breath. Certain foods will make your breath smell; don't eat pickled onions at lunchtime. Brush your teeth regularly. If you smoke, try to give it up.
- Hands and nails – both should be clean as the risk of spreading infection is then minimised. They should not be stained with hair colourant. Nails should not be bitten and should not be too long (dirt can get trapped underneath). Wear disposable gloves where necessary.
- Shoes – should be comfortable and allow feet to breathe. Leather shoes would be ideal. Cut down on foot odour by washing tights or socks frequently. Hair in the salon can harm the skin. It may

break the surface of the skin leaving the hairdresser open to risk of infection. The wearing of open toed shoes will increase the risk of infection.

- The skin – a bath or shower every day is essential because of the hot, humid atmosphere of the salon and the close contact the hairdresser has with the client. Always use deodorant or an antiperspirant (reduces underarm sweating). A little perfume is pleasant but too much can be overpowering.

Online activity 3.2 | **WWW**

Five in a row

3.2 Develop working relationships with colleagues

Team working is the key to a successful working environment and this success would not happen without your own input. All members of the team are needed. Make sure that you treat other members of the team with respect at all times. If you do not get on well with somebody outside work, you must still maintain a professional relationship at work. A friendly and approachable manner is essential for your own development within the team.

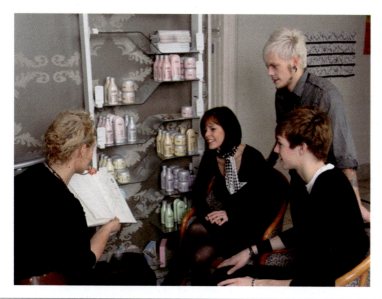

Figure 3.9 Working effectively as part of a team

 Key information

If you do not get on well with somebody outside work, you must still maintain a professional relationship at work.

Assisting others

Amongst other duties, you will be required to assist the stylists when they are carrying out a service. For example you may be asked to hold a client's hair in place whilst it is being styled or to pass foils/meshes during highlighting. Ensure that you are helpful to others whenever you are asked for assistance. Be quick to respond and do not be rude or feel that certain tasks are beneath you. Remember that your role in the team will change as you gain more experience.

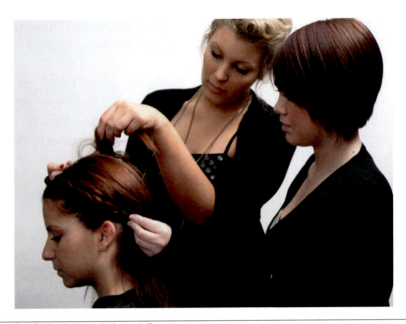

Figure 3.10 Assisting during styling

Definition

Assistance: To help.

Safety first

Never attempt a task that you have not been trained to do as this may put the safety of yourself and others at risk.

Asking for help

Never attempt a task that you have not been trained to do. This may put the safety of yourself and others at risk. When asking your colleagues for help or information, do it in a polite manner. It is important to treat others how you wish to be treated yourself.

Ensure you know the correct person to report to if you experience any problems in the salon. This will be a more senior member of staff in the salon.

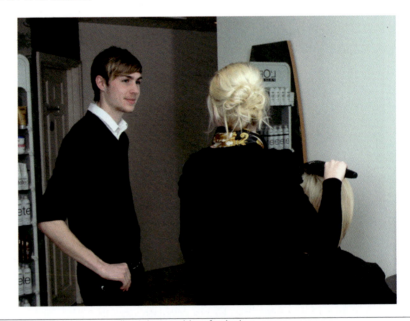

Figure 3.11 Always be polite when asking for help

WWW   **Online activity 3.3**

Round the board

3.3 Develop yourself within the job role

When you first start working in a salon as a trainee, your main job will be to help other members of staff in the salon. This is a great way of learning about all the treatments and services that your salon offers.

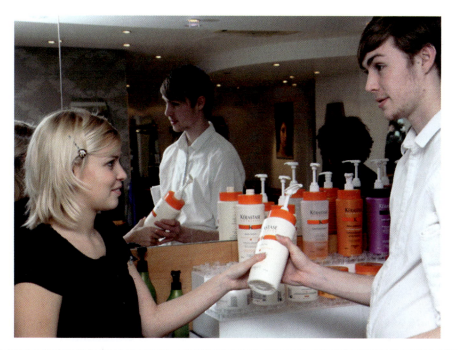

Figure 3.12 Helping others in the salon

Key information

You must remember to carry out your work to National Occupational Standards at all times. These standards make up your qualifications. If you do not do this it will greatly hinder the reputation of yourself and your salon.

If a task has been given to you by another member of staff, make sure that you ask them to explain if you are unclear about it. This is another way to ensure that the highest possible standard of service is given.

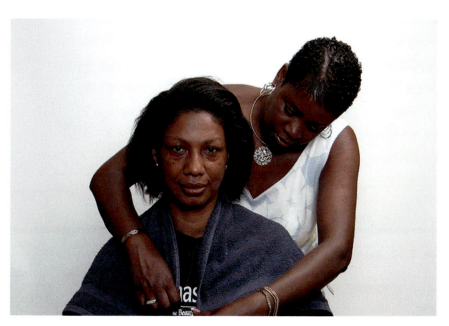

Figure 3.13 Ensure work is carried out to an acceptable standard at all times

Job description

Having a clear understanding of your role is essential for you to work effectively. You must make sure that you and your manager have the same defined role for your position. If you are confused in any way about part of your job, then speak to your manager to clarify any misunderstandings. When you start working in a salon, you will be given a job description. This is a written document outlining your:

- title
- the person to whom you are responsible
- location
- purpose
- duties
- standards needed.

Job Description

Job title:	Stylist
Responsible to:	Salon Manager
Based at:	The Hair Salon, Surrey
Purpose:	To provide services and treatments in the salon, whilst maintaining a high standard of customer care working in-line with company standards.
Duties:	Consult with clients, giving advice on services and treatments Provide high quality services and treatments to clients Give advice on products including aftercare Attend regular training sessions Assist salon manager Achieve performance targets set
Standards needed:	Ensure company policy is adhered to at all times

Figure 3.14 Job description

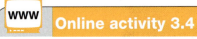

www **Online activity 3.4**

Select correct boxes

Appraisals

An appraisal is a system where yourself and your manager discuss your progress and personal contribution in the salon. Each salon will have its own staff appraisal system but you should have regular appraisals. Many salons will carry them out every three months.

It is not just about how you are doing in your role, but how you are developing as an individual. It should be thought of as a conversation between the two of you, not just your manager telling you how he or she feels about your work.

> **Key information**
>
> The appraisal process will identify:
>
> - what you have achieved
> - what you want to achieve
> - how to achieve it.

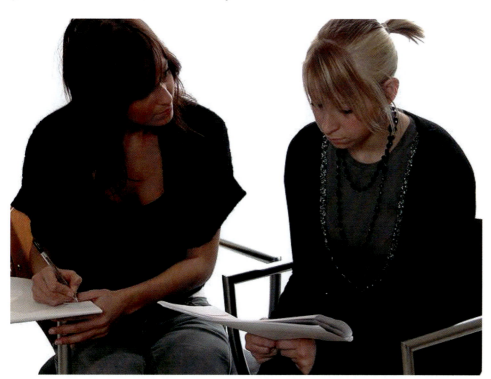

Figure 3.15 Appraisals are a two way conversation

Self-appraisal

Some companies will give a self-appraisal form for their staff to fill in and then a performance appraisal form that the employer will complete. This gives you a chance to discuss any points that you or your manager have made on your performance. It's not always easy to take a look at yourself so your manager should help by giving his or her opinion. Always listen to this opinion calmly even if you do not agree. Self-appraisal forms will contain whatever information your manager or salon manager feels is required for your position.

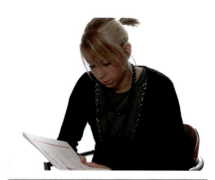

Figure 3.16 The employee fills in their own self-appraisal form

> **Key information**
>
> It's not always easy to take a look at yourself so your manager should help by giving his or her opinion. Always listen to this opinion calmly even if you do not agree.

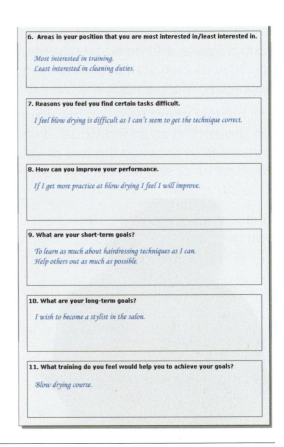

Self-appraisal

Name: *Sarah Jones*	Salon: *Cuts 4 U*
Position: *Trainee*	Age: *17*
Period covered: *Oct 2009 – Oct 2010*	Time in current position: *1 year*
Appraiser: *Karen McIntyre*	Date: *17th November*

1. What do you consider to be your main responsibilities?

Carrying out client care at all times.
Training in all aspects of hairdressing.
Assisting stylists.
Blow drying and shampooing.

2. Areas that you perform well.

I am good at shampooing and client care.

3. Areas that you could improve.

I find blow drying difficult at times and sometimes feel embarrassed to ask for help .

4. What do you feel have been your best achievements in your job role?

Winning 'Trainee' of the year in the salon awards..

5. Likes and dislikes about the company.

Likes – very happy team working.
Dislikes – sometimes I can't understand what the stylists are asking me to do, especially when it is busy on Saturdays.

6. Areas in your position that you are most interested in/least interested in.

Most interested in training.
Least interested in cleaning duties.

7. Reasons you feel you find certain tasks difficult.

I feel blow drying is difficult as I can't seem to get the technique correct.

8. How can you improve your performance.

If I get more practice at blow drying I feel I will improve.

9. What are your short-term goals?

To learn as much about hairdressing techniques as I can.
Help others out as much as possible.

10. What are your long-term goals?

I wish to become a stylist in the salon.

11. What training do you feel would help you to achieve your goals?

Blow drying course.

Figure 3.17 Sample self-appraisal

Strengths, weaknesses and targets

Part of the self-appraisal process will be to assess your own strengths and weaknesses. This will enable you to tackle any problem areas you may have. Be as honest as you can when establishing your strengths and weaknesses. You can see the strengths and weaknesses in Figure 3.17, the sample job appraisal. Sarah regards her strengths to be shampooing and client care whereas she regards her weakness as blow drying.

Short- and long-term goals

From your strengths and weaknesses you can set targets (i.e. short- and long-term goals that you wish to achieve). This helps to overcome any weaknesses you may have and shows that you are keen to learn. Your manager will then discuss these with you and can tell you whether he or she feels your short- and long-term goals are feasible. Figure 3.17 shows that Sarah's short-term goal is to improve her hairdressing techniques, which include blow drying, whereas her long-term goal is to become a stylist.

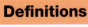

Definitions

Target: Objective set down for staff to reach.

Feasible: To be capable of being achieved.

www **Online activity 3.5**

Five in a row

Training and keeping skills up to date

You will notice on the self-appraisal form (Figure 3.17) that Sarah feels that to gain a full understanding of the principles of blow drying, she should take part in a training course. This is important throughout your career as a hairdresser as you must make sure your skills are kept up to date. You can do this not only through regular training, but also by attending hair shows, seminars and trade events.

Shadowing

Shadowing another member of staff is a great way to learn. If you get the opportunity to do this it will enable you to learn from somebody in the business with a greater amount of experience.

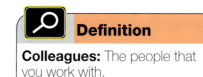

Key information

You can keep your skills up-to-date through regular training and by attending hair shows, seminars and trade events.

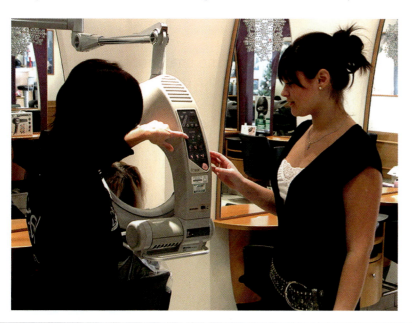

Figure 3.18 Shadowing another member of staff is a great way to learn

Asking others for help

In Sarah's appraisal (Figure 3.17) she wrote that she felt that she did not ask for help as much as she should. This is something she will need to tackle, as when you are training you will need to ask others for help on many different occasions. Other colleagues will understand that it is necessary for Sarah to ask for help so that she can be an effective member of staff.

Definition

Colleagues: The people that you work with.

Setting up a personal training plan

You can set up your own personal training plan by creating an action plan. Your long-term goal could be, for example, that in a year's time you want to complete your NVQ Level 1 in Hairdressing. You must break down the units that you wish to complete including the correct number of optional units.

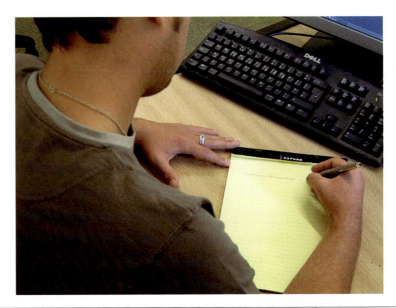

Figure 3.19 Set up a personal training plan

Let's say you wish to complete the shampooing/conditioning unit in one month's time. You should write down how you wish to achieve this. This may include:

- watch a junior shampooist – observe customer care
- listen to instructions – health and safety, salon security (looking after clients' belongings), how much shampoo to use (read manufacturer's instructions)
- learn about other products used in the salon
- practice on models until competent
- answer oral questions from other members of staff correctly
- complete assignments
- pass written question papers.

Review your training plan

The training plan is a guide enabling you to assess your progress. It should be reviewed and updated at regular periods to check that the objective or goal is being achieved.

Table 3.1 Example schedule

Areas	With help	Some help	Own work	Date
Shampoo		Yes		19/03
Condition		Yes		19/03
Blow dry	Yes			12/02

www Online activity 3.6

Select correct bars

Appeals and grievances

If you feel you have been treated unfairly, your salon will have a procedure for appeals and grievances. The first step would be to talk to a senior member of staff about the situation. If you cannot do this, then gain independent advice that can help you deal with the problem. If the issue is still not remedied, then the salon's process of appeals and grievances can be started.

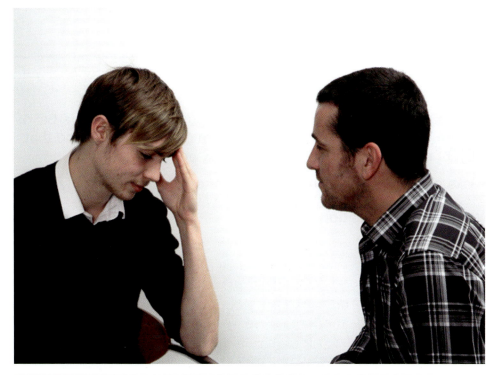

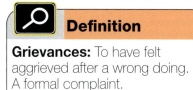
Definition

Grievances: To have felt aggrieved after a wrong doing. A formal complaint.

Figure 3.20 Talk to a more senior member of staff if you can

Now complete all the worksheets in the following section.

3

3.4 Worksheets

You can carry out these worksheets during your study of a chapter or unit, or at the end. If your college or training company is registered with ATT Training, lots more of these worksheets are available. Write your answers directly in the book – but only if you own it of course – if it is a library or college book, use a separate piece of paper!

Good communication

Good communication in the salon is always important, especially if a business is to succeed.

Communication can be in the following forms: verbal, non-verbal or written. You should be aware of your own communication and that of your clients in order to judge how they are feeling.

Make notes about the following types of communication:

Verbal communication

Non-verbal communication

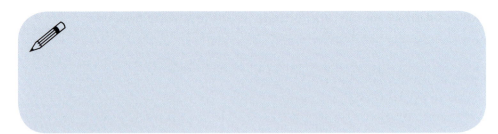

Written communication

Develop effective working relationships with colleagues

Read through the following text and fill in the gaps.

Team working is the key to a _____ working environment and this success would not happen without your own input. All members of the _____ are needed.

Make sure that you treat other members of the team with _____ at all times. If you do not get on well with somebody outside of work, you must still maintain a professional _____ inside work.

To develop yourself within the team, a _____ and _____ manner is essential.

Assisting others

Amongst other duties, you will be _____ to assist the stylists when they are carrying out a service. For example you may be asked to hold a _____ hair in place whilst it is being styled or to pass foils/meshes during highlighting.

Ensure that you are _____ to others whenever you are asked for assistance. Be _____ to respond and do not be rude or feel that certain tasks are beneath you. Remember that your role in the _____ will be changing as you gain more experience.

Asking for help

Never attempt a _____ that you have not been trained to do. This may put the safety of yourself and others at risk.

When asking your _____ for help or information, do it in a polite manner. It is important to treat others as you wish to be _____.

Ensure you know the correct person to _____ to if you experience any problems in the salon. This will be a more senior member of staff in the salon.

Setting yourself a personal training plan

You can create your own personal training plan by creating an action plan. Your long-term goal might be to complete your Hairdressing Level 2 qualification. You can then break that down to make your short-term goals by listing the units you want to complete (including the optional units).

Table 3.2 Example training plan

Areas	With help	Some help	Own work	Date
Shampoo		Yes		09/11
Condition		Yes		09/11
Blow dry	Yes			18/10

Now you should create your own training plan based on this.

3.5 Assessment

Well done! If you have studied all the content of this unit you may be ready to test your knowledge.

Check out the 'Preparing for assessments' section in Chapter 1 if you have not already done so. Always remember:

- You can only do your best if you have . . .
  - studied hard
  - completed the activities
  - completed the worksheets
  - practised, practised, practised
  - and then revised!

Now carry out the online multiple-choice quiz

. . . and good luck in the final exam, which will be arranged by your tutor/assessor.

Assist with salon reception duties

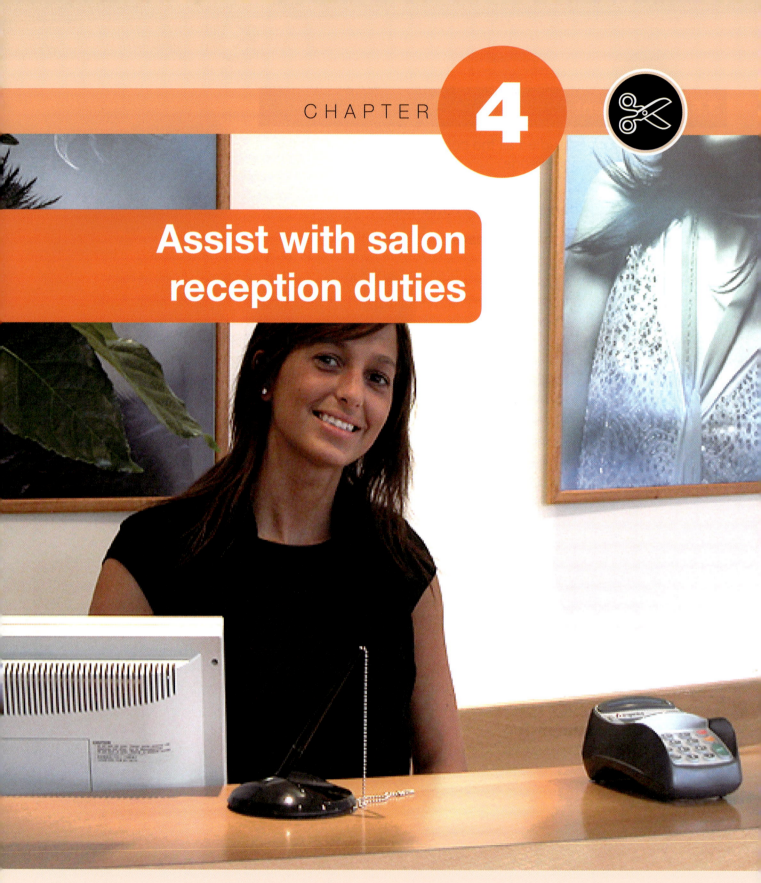

This chapter covers the NVQ/SVQ unit G2, Assist with salon reception duties

This chapter will help you to learn how to assist with salon reception duties. The reception area will be the first place that the client arrives and it is here they make appointments and pay for their services and treatments, so it is essential they gain a good impression.

In this chapter you will learn about:

■ maintaining the reception area

■ attending to clients and enquiries

■ helping to make appointments for salon services.

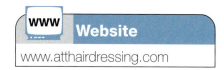

Website
www.atthairdressing.com

CHAPTER 4 ASSIST WITH SALON RECEPTION DUTIES: CONTENTS, SCREENS AND ACTIVITIES

Key:
Sections from the book are set in this colour
Screens available online are set in this colour
Online activity screens are set in this colour

4.1 Maintaining the reception area

The reception area should be maintained at all times to ensure that clients feel welcome as they enter the salon. Greeting the client in a warm and professional manner will also make the client feel at home. All parts of the reception should be kept clean and tidy, including stationery and retail products on display.

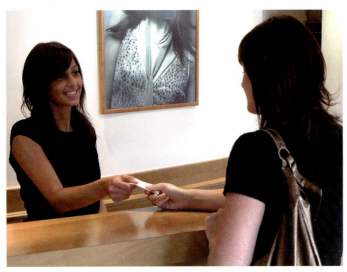

Figure 4.1 Clients should feel welcome in the reception area

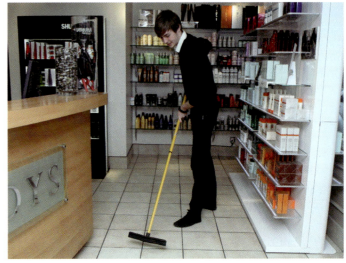

Figure 4.2 The reception area should be kept clean

Key information

The reception area should be maintained at all times, to ensure that clients feel welcome as they enter the salon.

Product checks

When checking the retail merchandise, look for product damage. It may be that the product is leaking, or the packaging may be damaged. Always check the sell-by date. If the product is damaged then you should remove it from display and report it to the relevant person. Also report any low levels of retail products.

Definitions

Retail: The sale of goods to the public.

Merchandise: Goods to be sold and bought.

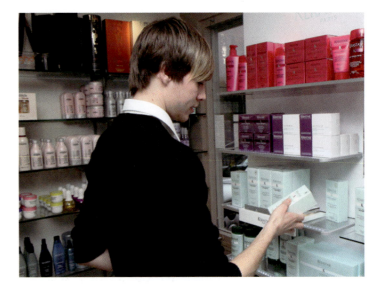

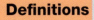
Figure 4.3 Check product condition

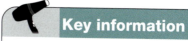
Stationery items

Stationery items to be kept at the reception are:

- service price lists
- product information leaflets
- appointment cards
- message pad
- appointment book
- promotional information or vouchers.

Online activity 4.1

Correct selection

Customer care

Whatever hospitality service your salon offers, make sure you follow it. You may or may not offer the client a drink on arrival, but you should always offer the client something to read. This could be a magazine or a style book.

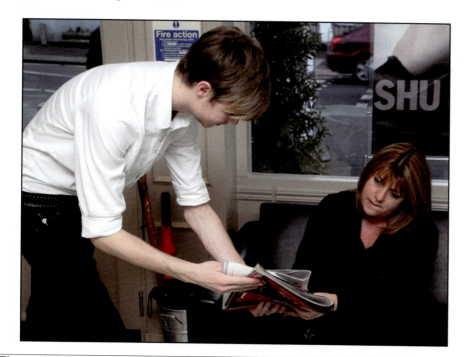

Figure 4.4 Always offer the client something to read

4.2 Attending to clients and enquiries

Whilst attending to clients and their enquiries, you must ensure that you are helpful and respectful at all times. Using successful communication will give out a professional image. Ensure that you suit your type of approach to the individual client you are speaking to. Always confirm what you understand to be the client's enquiry.

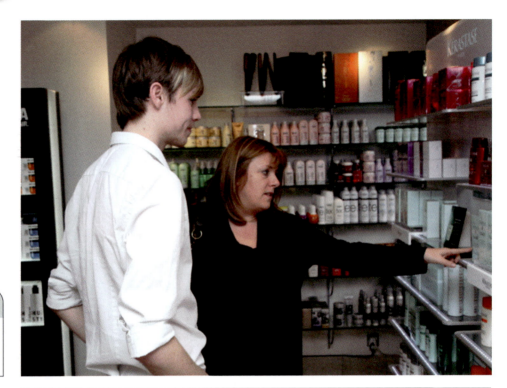

Figure 4.5 Ensure that you are helpful and respectful when dealing with enquiries

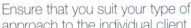

Key information

Ensure that you suit your type of approach to the individual client you are speaking to.

Checklist

Here is a checklist for you to follow:

- be friendly, have a pleasing smile
- be cheerful and enthusiastic, show interest and be alert
- be courteous when dealing with clients, using 'please' and 'thank you' as much as possible
- be efficient and well organised
- be quick, do not keep clients waiting
- be accurate, speak clearly, listen and try not to make mistakes
- develop different questioning skills using both open and closed questions. Questions that require a yes or no reply are known as closed questions. Using words such as when, who, what, if, etc., will enable the client to discuss their needs. This method is known as open questioning and is used to expand on what the client's wishes are, to help you to ensure a good service is provided.

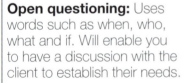

Key information

Open questioning: Uses words such as when, who, what and if. Will enable you to have a discussion with the client to establish their needs.

Closed questioning: Requires a 'yes' or 'no' answer.

Confirming appointments

As the client enters the salon, you should always confirm their appointment. Then you should ask them to take a seat. Do this in a polite manner. Then you should tell the stylist that their client has arrived. If the stylist is running late, you should tell the client so that they can decide what to do.

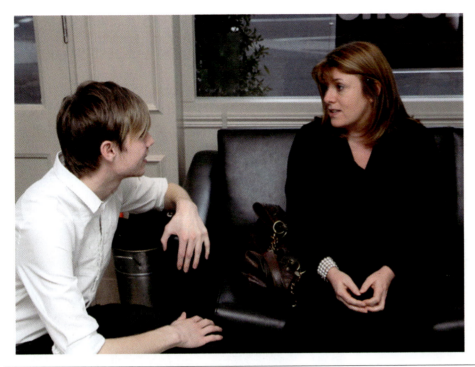

Figure 4.6 If the stylist is running late, then you should tell the client

🔍 **Definition**

Polite: To show regard to others. To use good manners.

Enquiries

Enquiries may be made by a variety of visitors, regular clients, new clients and casual clients. Some may have been recommended by other people and have knowledge about the salon, others may not. Enquiries that you will deal with will be either face-to-face or on the telephone.

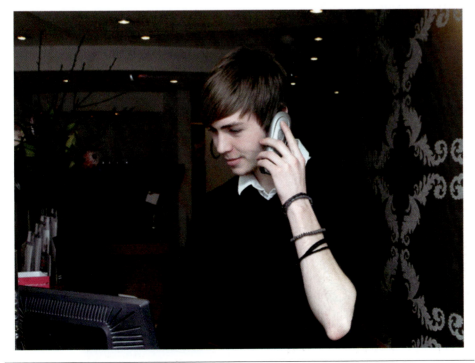

Figure 4.7 Telephone enquiry

Dealing with enquiries

When dealing with an enquiry it is essential to establish the purpose of the enquiry and the information required. All messages should be recorded accurately and completely. They should then be passed on promptly to the correct person. You must have knowledge of the products and services sold in the salon (e.g. cost of products and treatments) as well as the time required.

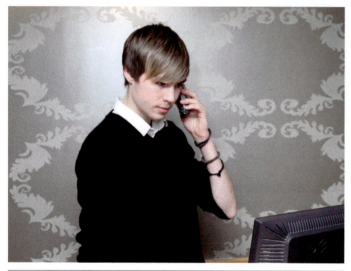

Figure 4.8 Pass on messages . . .

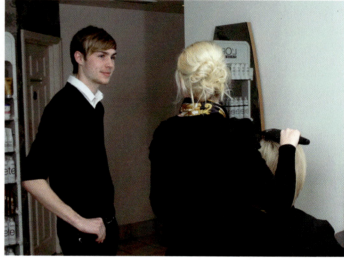

Figure 4.9 . . . promptly

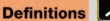

Definitions 🔍
Accurate: Exact.
Promptly: Straight away.

WWW **Online activity 4.2**
Round the board

Referring enquiries

Sometimes you may not be able to deal with an enquiry either face-to-face or on the telephone. If this is the case, make sure you know the correct person to refer the issue to. Do this quickly so that action can be taken immediately.

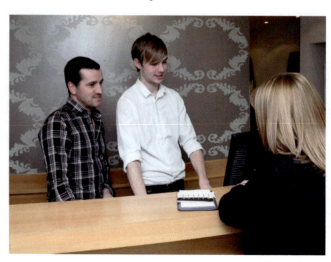

Figure 4.10 Refer enquiries to your manager if you need help

Taking telephone messages

You will be required to take messages. The details should be recorded clearly and the following points should be observed when taking a message:

- identify the name of the salon to the caller
- state your own name
- enquire who is calling
- write the telephone number of the caller
- note the company who the caller represents
- note whether or not the message is urgent
- the name of the person to whom the message should be given
- who recorded the message.

Giving out confidential information

This should only be given out to those who are authorised (i.e. salon owner, managers or staff). If information is not kept confidential then the Data Protection Act will be breached. This may result in you losing your position at the salon.

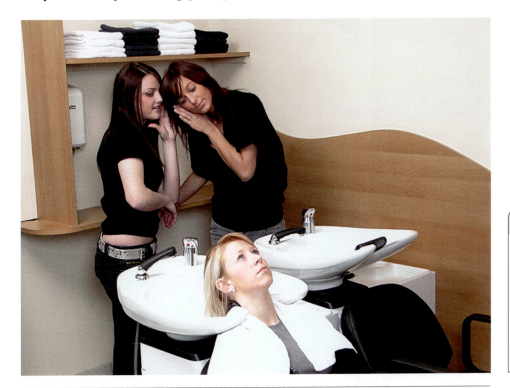

Figure 4.11 You should never gossip about clients in this way

> **🔍 Definition**
>
> **Data Protection Act:**
> A United Kingdom Act of Parliament which defines UK law on the processing of data on identifiable living people. It is the main piece of legislation governing the protection of personal data in the UK.

Online activity 4.3   **www**

Five in a row

Appointment system

Appointments are made over the telephone or face to face. They must be taken correctly and straight away. As you are helping with these appointments, it is essential that you are aware of the services that your salon offers.

To ensure the efficient running of the salon the appointment system must be well organised. Each salon will have its own system for making appointments, with many using a computerised system.

Some salons use an appointment book and divide it into columns with the stylist's name at the top and the times down the side.

Whichever system is used, it is recommended that the following points should be recorded: date, client's name, telephone number, the time, service required and the member of staff responsible for the scheduled service. The details entered should be pencilled in so that any alterations are easily made.

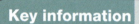
Key information

Whichever appointment system is used in your salon, you must make a note of the:

- date
- client's name
- client's telephone number
- scheduled appointment time
- service required
- member of staff responsible for service.

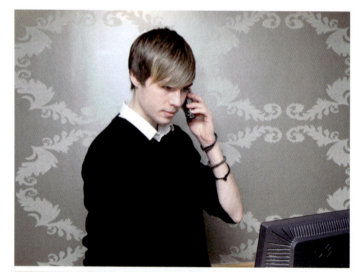

Figure 4.12 Appointments can be by telephone

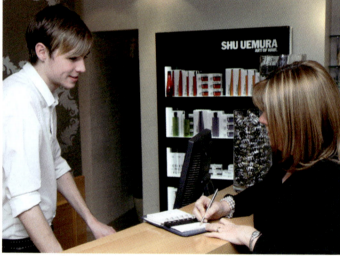

Figure 4.13 Appointments can be made in person

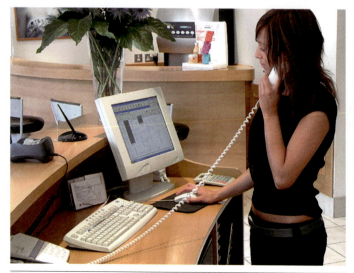

Figure 4.14 A computerised system

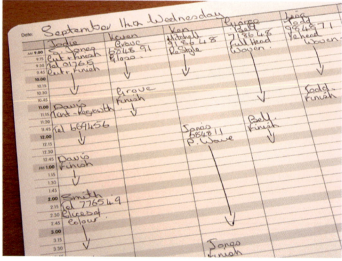

Figure 4.15 A typical appointment book

Online activity 4.4

Select correct boxes

Asking for assistance

If you are unsure about anything when recording appointments you should ask for help. It may be that you need to ask the stylist concerned if it is a very complex appointment, or it is difficult for you to schedule in. If the client is booking in person, the stylist may need to look at the client's hair to see how long they will need to carry out the service. If a client looks unhappy about something, you should ask them to take a seat and then find a more senior staff member to talk to them about the problem.

⚠ Safety first

The stylist may need to look at the client's hair to see how long they will need to carry out a service.

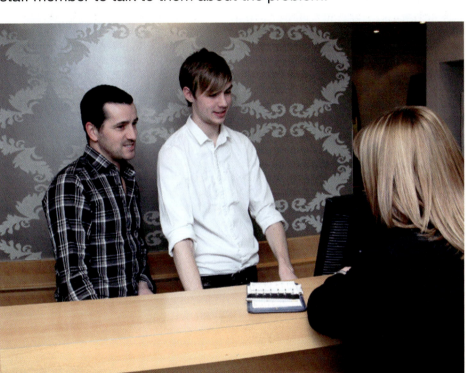

Figure 4.16 Ask a senior member of staff for help if necessary

Confirming appointments

When the client has made his or her next appointment in person, the details (time, service, date and stylist) should be entered onto an appointment card. This should then be handed to the client. You should thank the client for their custom and verbally confirm the next appointment. If appointments are made over the phone, repeat the details back to the client so that these can be confirmed.

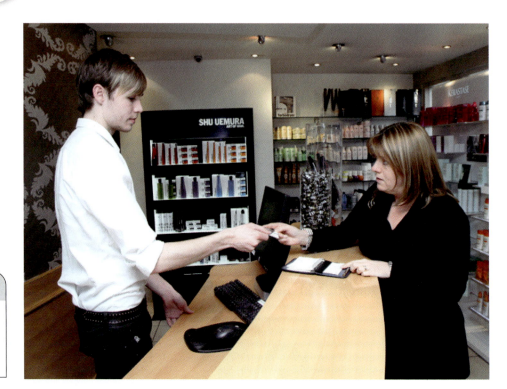

Figure 4.17 Verbally confirm the client's appointment

Now complete all the worksheets in the following section.

Key information

If appointments are made over the phone, repeat the details back to the client so that these can be confirmed.

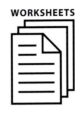

4.3 Worksheets

You can carry out these worksheets during your study of a chapter or unit, or at the end. If your college or training company is registered with ATT Training, lots more of these worksheets are available. Write your answers directly in the book – but only if you own it of course – if it is a library or college book, use a separate piece of paper!

Customer care

All salons will offer hospitality services to their clients.

What are the hospitality procedures in your salon? Do you offer clients refreshments? Make detailed notes here:

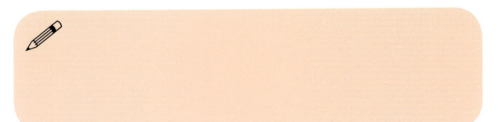

Do you think these hospitality services can be improved in any way? What else would you offer your clients? Make notes here:

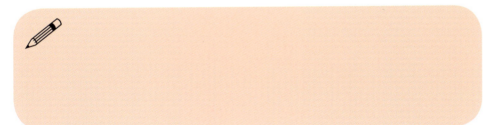

Confirming appointments

As the client enters the salon, you should always confirm their appointment.

What is your salon's policy for confirming customer appointments when they arrive at the salon? Make a list of each of the steps that you would follow to complete this process:

1.

2.

3.

4.

5.

6.

7.

8.

9.

10.

Taking telephone messages

You will be required to take messages. The details should be recorded clearly and the following points should be observed when taking a message:

- identify the name of the salon to the caller
- state your own name
- inquire who is calling
- write the telephone number of the caller
- note the company that the caller represents
- the date and time of the call
- whether or not the message is urgent
- the name of the person to whom the message should be given
- who recorded the message.

Working with a partner, practise answering the telephone and taking messages. Person 1 should be the customer to begin with, then you should swap round so that Person 2 takes the role of the customer. Make any notes that you might find useful here:

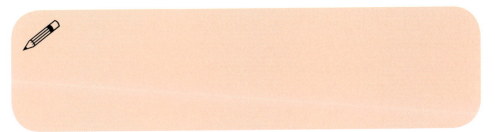

4.4 Assessment

Well done! If you have studied all the content of this unit you may be ready to test your knowledge.

Check out the 'Preparing for assessments' section in Chapter 1 if you have not already done so and always remember:

- You can only do your best if you have . . .
  - studied hard
  - completed the activities
  - completed the worksheets
  - practised, practised, practised
  - and then revised!

 Now carry out the online multiple-choice quiz

. . . and good luck in the final exam, which will be arranged by your tutor/ assessor.

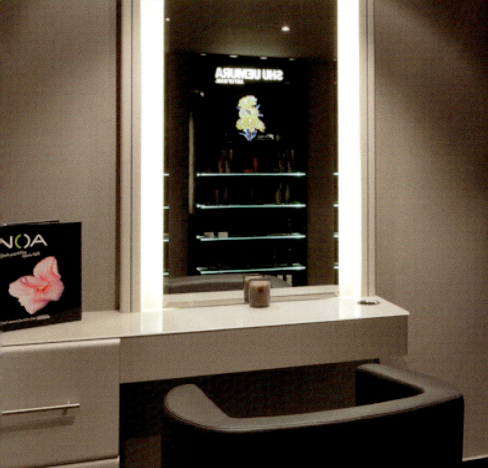

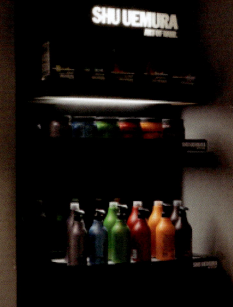

Prepare for hair services and maintain work areas

This chapter covers the NVQ/SVQ unit GH3, Prepare for hair services and maintain work areas

Keeping the salon or barber's shop clean and tidy is essential at all times. This will keep everyone in the salon safe. The responsibility for ensuring this happens will be on everybody in the working environment.

In this chapter you will learn about:

- preparing for hair services
- maintaining the work area for hair services.

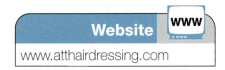

Website www.atthairdressing.com

CHAPTER 5 PREPARE FOR HAIR SERVICES AND MAINTAIN WORK AREAS: CONTENTS, SCREENS AND ACTIVITIES

Key:
Sections from the book are set in this colour
Screens available online are set in this colour
Online activity screens are set in this colour

5.1 Preparing for hair services

You will be responsible for helping stylists and barbers by:

- preparing their materials, tools and equipment
- ensuring that these materials, tools and equipment are prepared in time
- ensuring all tools are clean and sterile
- getting client records ready for stylists' consultations.

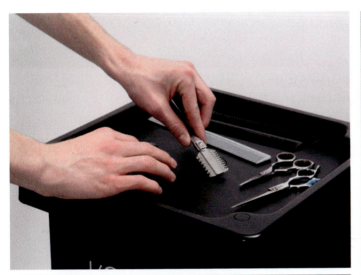

Figure 5.1 Preparing tools and equipment

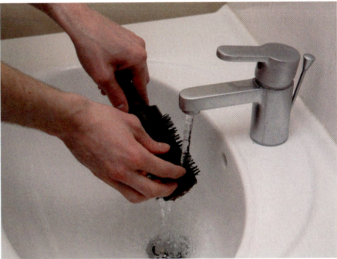

Figure 5.2 Ensure tools and equipment are clean and sterile

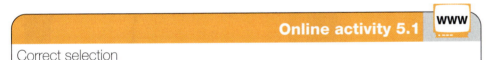

Online activity 5.1 WWW

Correct selection

Definition

Sterile: Free from disease-causing micro-organisms.

Materials, tools and equipment

You will be required to set up materials, tools and equipment. You should consider what the stylist might need for their service. The following may need to be prepared prior to the stylist or barber commencing their service:

- brushes, combs and neck brush
- perming equipment including rollers, end papers and section clips
- colouring equipment including bowls, brushes, meshes or foils
- towels and gowns
- heated styling equipment.

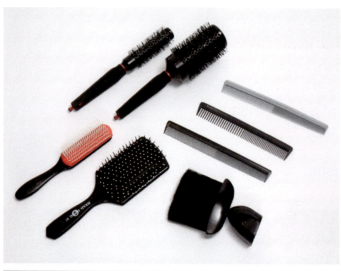

Figure 5.3 Brushes, combs and neck brush

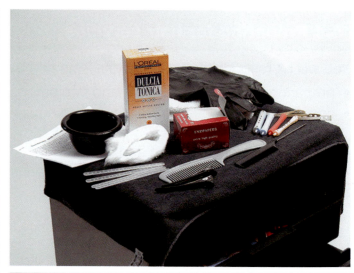

Figure 5.4 Perming equipment including rollers, end papers and section clips

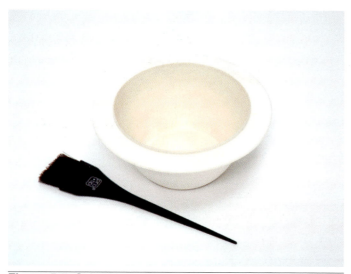

Figure 5.5 Colouring equipment

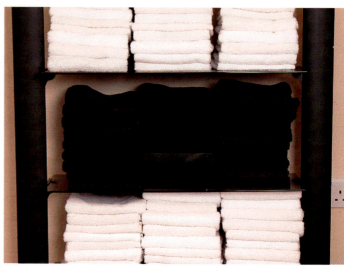

Figure 5.6 Towels and gowns

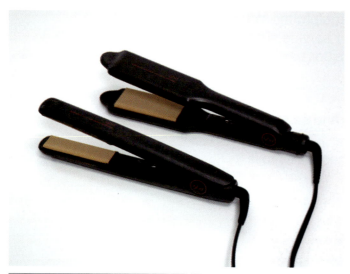

Figure 5.7 Heated styling equipment

Setting up trolleys

Trolleys must be set up prior to the client arriving. You may need to organise this many times during the day. The stylist or barber will tell you what service they will be carrying out and then you must set the trolley up accordingly. Remember that perm and setting rollers will be colour-coded according to size. Stylists may ask you to prepare the rollers explaining the colour they wish to have.

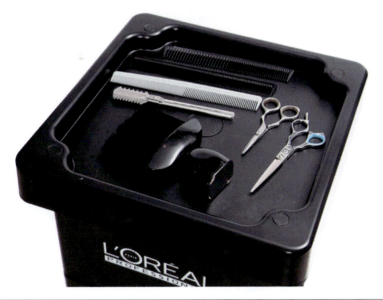

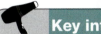
Key information

The stylist or barber will tell you what service they will be carrying out and then you must set the trolley up accordingly.

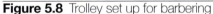

Figure 5.8 Trolley set up for barbering

Setting up materials, tools and equipment on time

Timing is very important when preparing materials, tools and equipment. The stylist or barber cannot be kept waiting. They must have everything they need to carry out the service at the agreed time.

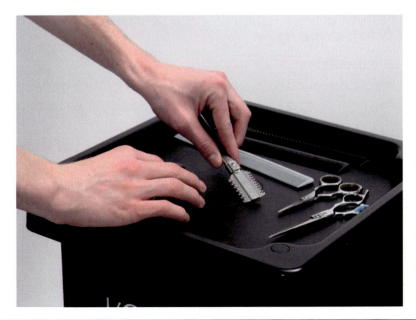

Figure 5.9 Everything required by the stylist must be on the trolley

Ensuring tools and equipment are clean and sterile

Bacteria will breed in the right conditions and this is why not just the salon, but all tools and equipment must be kept clean at all times. Brushes and combs should be washed in hot soapy water and then sterilised. Perm rods, setting rollers and colouring equipment (i.e. brushes and combs) should also be washed in hot soapy water before sterilising. If any tools are accidently dropped on the floor, then they should be re-washed and sterilised. Trolleys can be cleaned with a disinfectant spray and cloth.

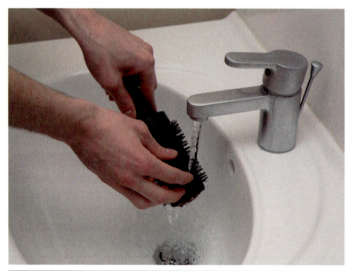

Figure 5.10 Brushes and combs should be washed in hot soapy water and then sterilised

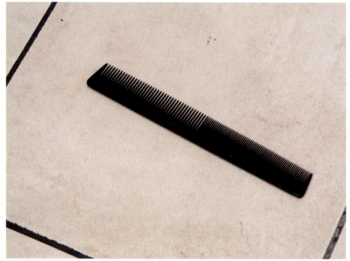

Figure 5.11 Re-wash and sterilse any items dropped on the floor

Methods of sterilisation

Salons may use a variety of ways to sterilise equipment (make free of micro-organisms). Remember to always wash brushes and combs before sterilising.

Autoclave (heat)

This is the recommended method of sterilisation for small metal items. The high temperature steam produced destroys all micro-organisms.

UV cabinet (ultraviolet radiation)

Clean tools can be stored in a UV cabinet once they have been sterilised.

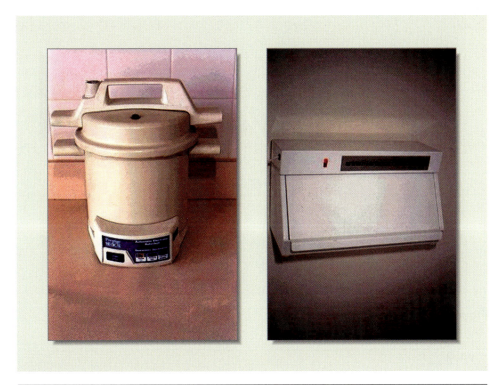

Figure 5.12 Autoclave and UV cabinet

Chemical sterilisation

Proprietary sterilising solutions and sprays are available for sterilising equipment. To be effective the chemical solutions should be used for the correct length of time and mixed according to the manufacturers' instructions.

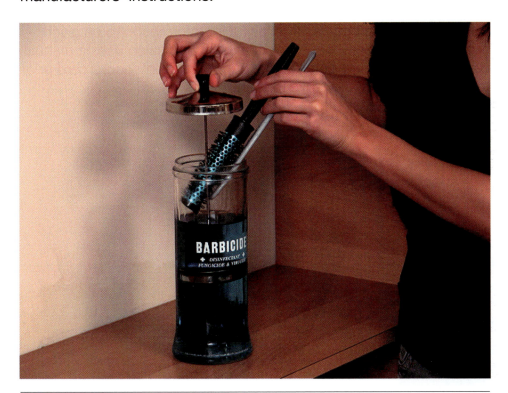

Figure 5.13 Chemical sterilising solution

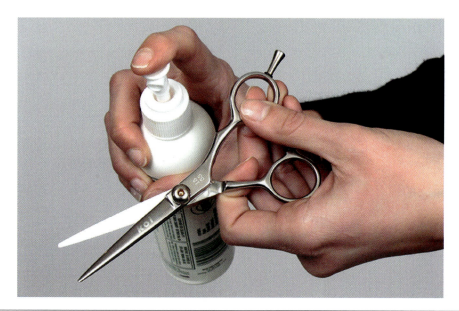

Figure 5.14 Sterilising sprays can be used for cleaning scissors and clippers

WWW **Online activity 5.2**

Check it

Definition

Data Protection Act: An Act of Parliament which defines UK law on the processing of data on identifiable living people. It is the main piece of legislation that governs the protection of personal data in the UK.

Key information

If your salon uses a manual card system for client details, take out the relevant record card prior to the consultation and leave it ready for the stylist.

Client records

Client records detailing all the tests, services and treatments that they have are kept in the salon. This will enable all staff to gain knowledge of this information. They can be kept on a computer system or on record cards. All client records are confidential. The Data Protection Act makes it unlawful for information to be given out in regards to personal client details. If your salon uses a manual card system for client details, take out the relevant record card prior to the consultation and leave it ready for the stylist.

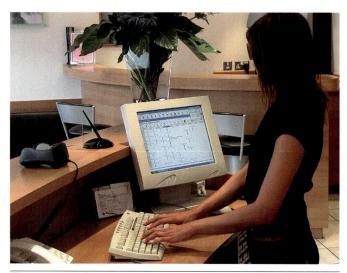

Figure 5.15 Client records are stored on computer systems

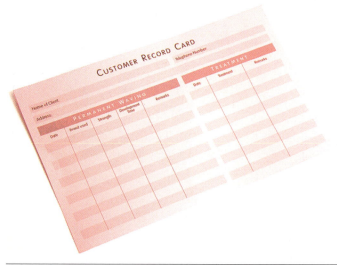

Figure 5.16 Client records can also be kept on manual record cards

5.2 Maintaining work areas for hair services

To maintain the work area you should know the correct methods of keeping everything clean and tidy in the salon.

Waste material disposal

Covered waste bins which contain a polythene bin liner should be used for everyday items of salon waste (including hair clippings, disposable capes etc.). These should either be emptied daily or when full. Razor blades and any other sharp items should be kept away from general salon waste and placed in a safe closed container before disposal. Chemical waste should be kept away from general waste. Any contaminated waste should be put in a separate bag and disposed of immediately.

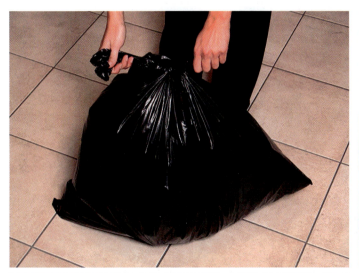

Figure 5.17 Polythene bin liners should be used for salon waste

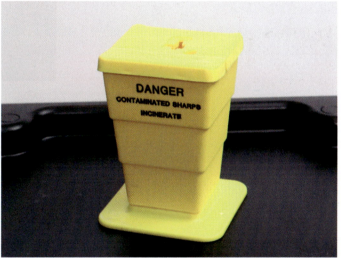

Figure 5.18 Sharps boxes are used to dispose of razors

Control of Substances Hazardous to Health Regulations 2002

These are commonly called the COSHH regulations. These lay down the essential requirements for controlling exposure to hazardous substances and for protecting people who may be affected by them.

A substance is considered to be hazardous if it can cause harm to the body. It only poses a risk if it is:

- inhaled (breathed in)
- in contact with the skin
- absorbed through the skin
- injected into the body
- introduced into the body via cuts etc.

For more information about the COSHH regulations see Chapter 2.

Cleaning and checking work equipment – basins and backwashes

Basins and backwashes should be cleaned and checked at the start of every day and after every use. A spray cleaner can be used for cleaning.

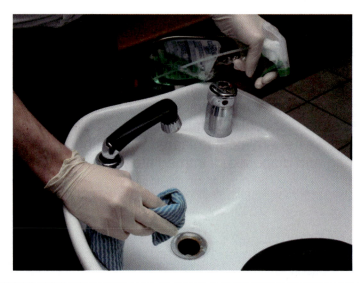

Figure 5.19 Cleaning a basin

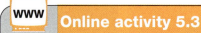

Cleaning equipment used for added heat

When cleaning hood dryers and other equipment used for added heat, take care as they all run with electricity. See Chapter 2 for more information. Use a recommended product (e.g. a spray cleaner). Clean and dust them at the start of every day and throughout the day.

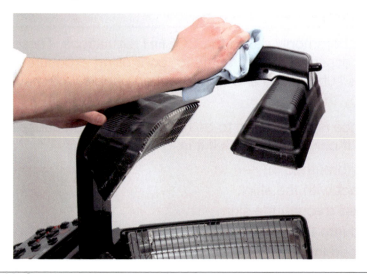

Figure 5.20 Cleaning equipment used for adding heat

Towels and gowns

The salon must never run out of clean towels and gowns and it may be your responsibility to make sure this does not happen. There will be constant need for washing and tumble drying these, so make sure you know how to use the electrical equipment.

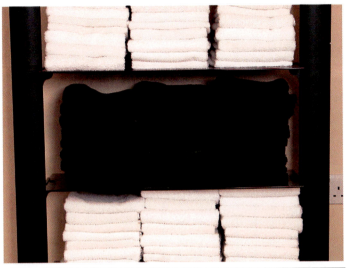

Figure 5.21 Clean towels

Figure 5.22 Always use a clean gown

Replenishing stock levels

You will be responsible for keeping products replenished in the salon. You will need to do this continually throughout the day, so make sure you check the products (i.e. colour, shampoo and conditioner) by the basins and also the items on display for sale.

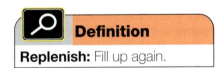

Definition

Replenish: Fill up again.

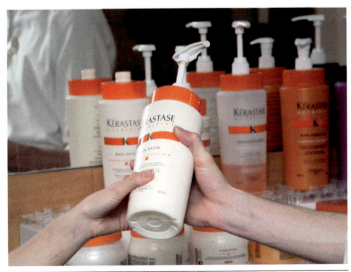

Figure 5.23 Check the products by the basins

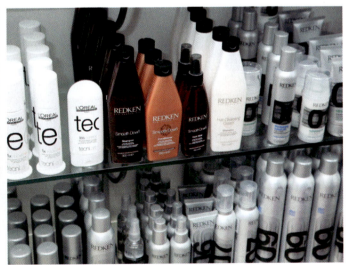

Figure 5.24 Check the display items

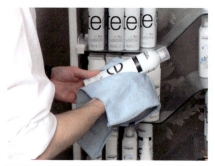

Figure 5.25 Topping up a shampoo dispenser

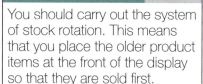

Figure 5.26 Dust the products to ensure displays look appealing

> ### Key information
>
> You should carry out the system of stock rotation. This means that you place the older product items at the front of the display so that they are sold first.

Replenishing shampoo and conditioners

To top up the bulk size dispenser shampoo and conditioners, you should first of all ask to take them away into the stock area. Then take off the screw top. You must then clean the pump and place the new product into the dispenser. Only fill up to just below the neck. This stops any product being wasted. If you notice any other styling resources running low, you should ask if you should replace it.

Replenishing retail display

If products on the retail display run low, this can result in a loss of sales. Therefore it is important to keep them filled up at all times. You may be asked to help out the receptionist by doing this. Always ask before fetching the replacements for the display. Before placing out the new items, clean the products that are currently there by dusting. Displays should always look clean and appealing to the customer. Carry out the system of stock rotation. This means that you place the older product items at the front of the display so that they are sold first.

> **www** **Online activity 5.4**
>
> Five in a row

Keeping equipment, materials and records in their place

Make sure that when you have taken something to clean or check, that it is placed back in the correct place. This will ensure that they are not lost in the salon.

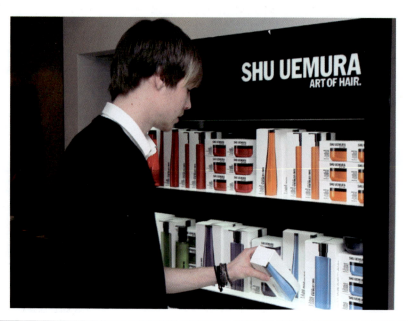

Figure 5.27 Ensure items are placed back where you found them

Cleaning work surfaces

All work surfaces should be cleaned thoroughly. This must be done at the beginning of each day and after every client. All cups, saucers, magazines and tools must be tidied away. The surface should be left in a suitable condition for the next service to begin.

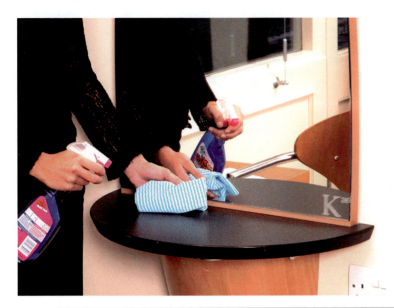

Figure 5.28 Cleaning work surfaces

Floors

Floors should be kept clean; hair clippings should be swept up to prevent disease and accidents. If any spillages occur they will need to be mopped up then and there. If you do not know what the spillage is, then you must ask somebody who does. If floors are wet, notices should be left to warn clients and other staff. Ensure that you use the correct cleaning products when cleaning the floor. Read the manufacturer's instructions before use and wear the correct PPE.

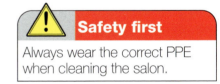
Safety first

Always wear the correct PPE when cleaning the salon.

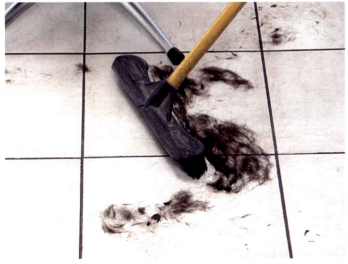

Figure 5.29 Sweep up hair clippings

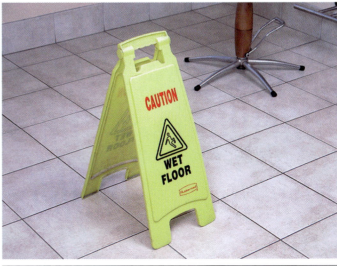

Figure 5.30 Warn clients and other staff members if the floor is wet

Salon chairs and mirrors

Keep salon chairs clean and free of hair. Dust and clean the base of the chair. Mirrors should be cleaned before the clients arrive and throughout the day. A spray cleaner can be used to do this.

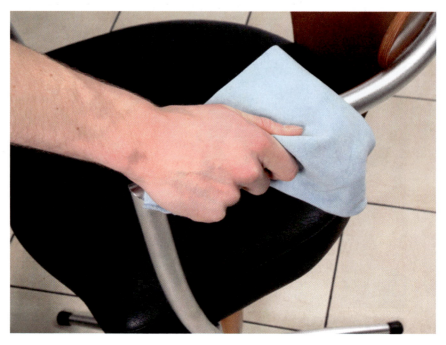

Figure 5.31 Clean the salon chairs

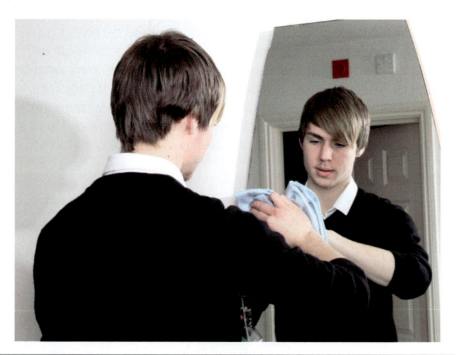

Figure 5.32 Mirrors should be cleaned throughout the day

www   Online activity 5.5

Wordsearch

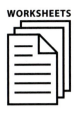

5.3 Worksheets

WORKSHEETS

You can carry out these worksheets either during your study of a chapter or unit, or at the end. If your college or training company is registered with ATT Training, lots more of these worksheets are available. Write your answers directly in the book – but only if you own it of course – if it is a library or college book, use a separate piece of paper!

Client records

Answer these questions about the records that should be kept on all clients:

1. What information will be included in the client records?

2. Why are client records important to assist the hairdresser?

3. How are client records kept?

4. Client records are confidential. True or false?

5. What is the name of the Act that makes it unlawful for client's personal information to be released?

6. When should you consult the client records – before, during or after the service?

Waste material disposal

Covered waste bins which contain a polythene bin liner should be used for everyday items of salon waste (including hair clippings, disposable capes etc.). These should be emptied daily or when full. Razor blades and any other sharp items should be kept away from general salon waste and placed in a safe closed container before disposal. Chemical waste should be kept away from general waste. Any contaminated waste should be put in a separate bag and disposed of immediately.

Now answer the following questions about what the procedures are in your salon:

1. Who is responsible for emptying the covered waste bins (which contain polythene bin liners)?

2. Where is the closed container that is used to dispose of razor blades kept in your salon?

3. Who is responsible for emptying the safe box used to dispose of razor blades?

4. Where should the safe box used to dispose of razor blades be emptied?

5. What would be considered contaminated waste?

6. What is the procedure for disposing of contaminated waste?

Ensuring tools and equipment are clean and sterile

Answer the following questions about tools and equipment in the salon:

1. What will breed in the right conditions?

2. How should brushes and combs be washed?

3. How should perm rods and setting equipment be washed?

4. How should colouring equipment be washed?

5. What should you do if you accidently drop any tools on the floor?

6. How should trolleys be cleaned?

7. How often should trolleys be cleaned?

5.4 Assessment

Well done! If you have studied all the content of this unit you may be ready to test your knowledge.

Check out the 'Preparing for assessments' section in Chapter 1 if you have not already done so, and always remember:

- You can only do your best if you have . . .
  - studied hard
  - completed the activities
  - completed the worksheets
  - practised, practised, practised
  - and then revised!

 Now carry out the online multiple-choice quiz

. . . and good luck in the final exam, which will be arranged by your tutor/assessor.

Shampoo and condition hair

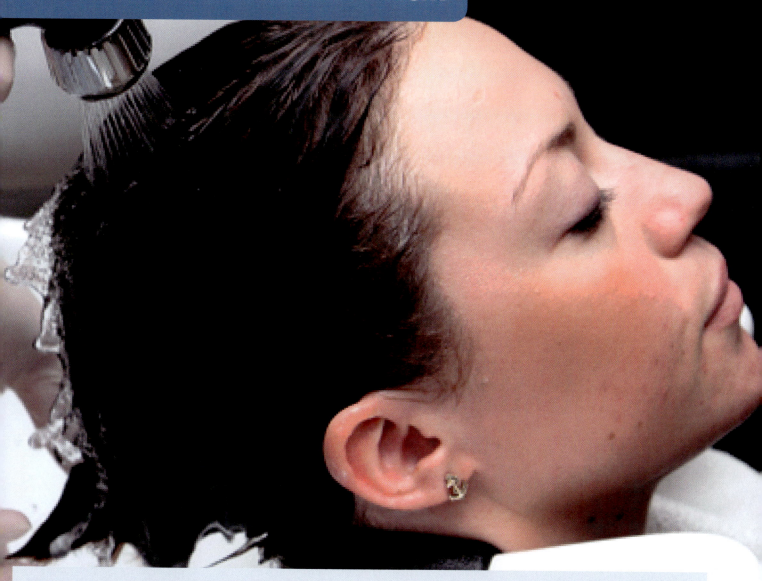

This chapter covers the NVQ/SVQ unit GH1, *Shampoo and condition hair*

This chapter shows you the techniques used for shampooing and conditioning the hair. Instructions from the stylist should be followed at all times.

In this chapter you will learn about:

- maintaining effective and safe methods of working when shampooing and conditioning hair
- shampooing hair
- applying conditioners to hair.

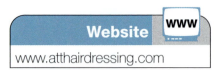

CHAPTER 6 SHAMPOO AND CONDITION HAIR: CONTENTS, SCREENS AND ACTIVITIES

Key:
Sections from the book are set in this colour
Screens available online are set in this colour
Online activity screens are set in this colour

Working safely

Introduction	Dermatitis
Safety when shampooing, conditioning and treating	Electricity at Work Regulations 1989
Prepare client for service	Correct selection
Round the board	Products
Client comfort at the basin	Removing waste after shampooing and conditioning
Correct posture	Suggested service times
COSHH	

Shampoo hair

Introduction	Client care
PH, acidity and alkalinity	Round the board
Shampooing products	Shampooing procedure 1
Types of shampoos and ingredients	Shampooing procedure 2
Scrambled words	Shampooing procedure 3
Purpose of the shampoo	Shampooing procedure 4
How shampoos work	Drag Into correct order
Massage techniques	

Condition hair and scalp

Introduction	Five in a row
Types of conditioners	Application of conditioners 1
Surface conditioners	Application of conditioners 2
Treatment conditioners	Worksheet – Dermatitis
Tools and equipment	Worksheet – How shampoo works
Massage techniques	Worksheet – Types of conditioner

6.1 Working safely

This section covers the health and safety issues concerned with shampooing and conditioning the hair.

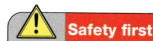

Safety first

Chapter 2 covers health and safety working methods in more detail. Refer to this unit if needed.

Prepare client for service

Help the client to put on a gown to protect his or her clothing while in the salon. Always use fresh, clean and sterile towels and use a new gown for each client.

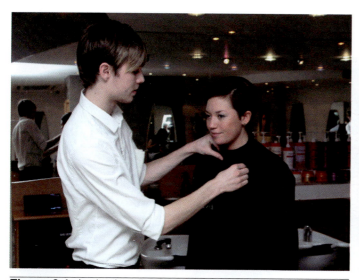

Figure 6.1 Assist the client to put on a gown

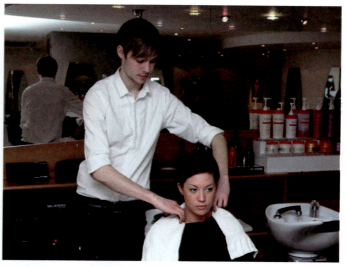

Figure 6.2 Always use fresh, clean towels

Ask the client to remove any jewellery that may interfere with the service, for example large loop earrings or heavy chains around the neck. Offer physical support if necessary to an incapacitated or infirm client. Ensure that there are no obstacles or hazards in the way. The stylist will select a suitable shampoo and conditioner.

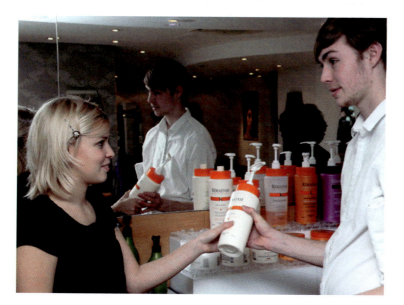

Figure 6.3 The stylist will tell you which shampoo and conditioner to use

www   Online activity 6.1

Round the board

Client comfort at the basin

If you are using a forward-facing basin offer the client a face cloth or a folded towel to protect the eyes during the service. When using a backwash basin, manoeuvre or support the client's head over the basin. Make sure that the client's neck feels comfortable at all times. Towels should be below the basin neckline. This prevents water seeping into the towels and soaking the client's clothes.

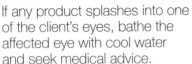

Safety first

If any product splashes into one of the client's eyes, bathe the affected eye with cool water and seek medical advice.

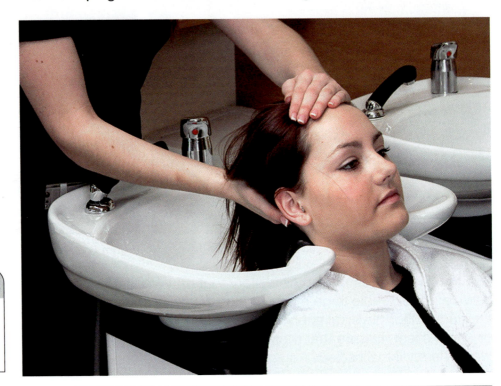

Figure 6.4 Supporting the client's head

Correct posture

When standing at the washbasin, stand with your weight evenly distributed throughout your body. Wear flat, comfortable shoes as this will help weight distribution. Do not bend over the basins, extend the arms from the shoulders. Do not lean across the client – walk around to the other side and work. All of these points help to minimise the effects of bad posture on the body. The most common effect of a bad posture is fatigue.

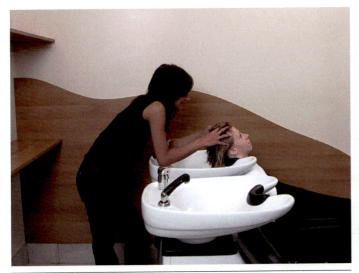

Figure 6.5 Incorrect posture

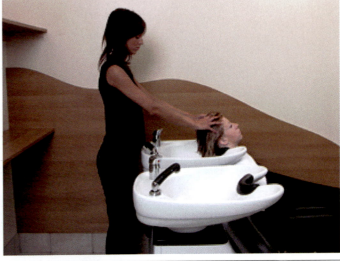

Figure 6.6 Correct posture

Control of Substances Hazardous to Health Regulations 2002 (COSHH)

These are commonly called the COSHH Regulations and they lay down the essential requirements for controlling exposure to hazardous substances and for protecting people who may be affected by them. A substance is considered to be hazardous if it can cause harm to the body. It only poses a risk if it is:

- inhaled (breathed in)
- ingested (swallowed)
- in contact with the skin
- absorbed through the skin
- injected into the body or
- introduced into the body via cuts etc.

For more information about the COSHH Regulations refer to Chapter 2.

Dermatitis

This is a very common skin disease in hairdressers and is caused by hands regularly being exposed to certain products and carrying out wet-work. Dermatitis can be prevented by:

- ensuring shampoo and conditioner are rinsed from your hands
- drying hands thoroughly
- moisturising regularly
- wearing disposable gloves.

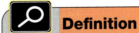 **Definition**

Fatigue: Tiredness can be caused by poor working posture.

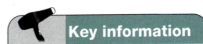 **Key information**

Dermatitis is a very common skin disease in hairdressers and is caused by hands being regularly exposed to certain products and carrying out wet-work.

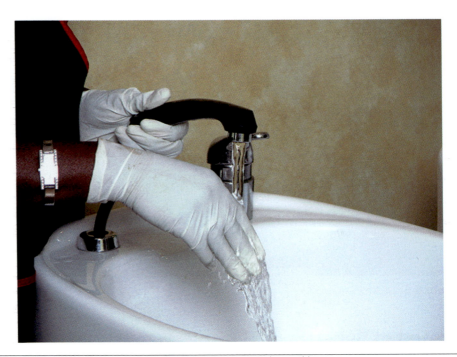

Figure 6.7 Using disposable gloves can prevent dermatitis

Electricity at Work Regulations 1989

These regulations state that you must:

- Always check electrical equipment before using. Look for loose wires and ensure that the plug is not cracked or damaged in any way. Check that the cord is not frayed or cracked.
- Never use electrical equipment with wet hands.
- Electrical equipment should be maintained regularly and checked by a suitably qualified person. Once checked, the equipment should have a certificate or label acknowledging it.
- Faulty electrical equipment in the workplace must be removed, labelled as faulty and reported to the relevant person.

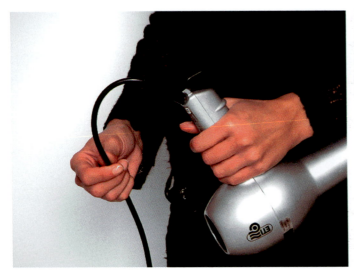

Figure 6.8 Checking electrical equipment for damage

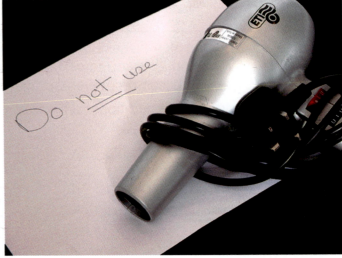

Figure 6.9 Correct labelling of faulty equipment

Online activity 6.2 www

Correct selection

Products

Make sure that you read manufacturers' instructions before using products. If you notice that products are running low, ensure that you inform the relevant person according to your salon's policy. Do this without delay as running out of stock would have negative consequences for your salon's reputation. Equally, do not waste products as this will not be cost effective for the salon.

> ⚠️ **Safety first**
>
> Make sure that you read the manufacturers' instructions before using any products.

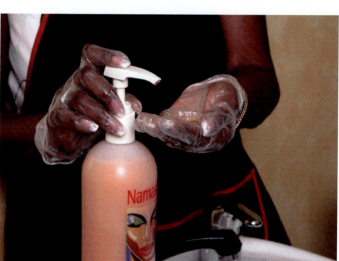

Figure 6.10 Keep a check on products as you use them

Removing waste after shampooing and conditioning

After shampooing and conditioning the hair, ensure that the basin is left clean ready for the next client. Check the plug is free of hair as this will block the sink.

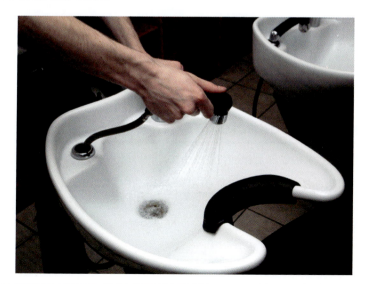

Figure 6.11 Rinse out the basin after shampooing and conditioning

Suggested service times

Commercially viable times for shampooing, conditioning and/or treating hair are as follows (excluding any development times):

Table 5.1 Suggested service times

Length of hair	Time
Above shoulders	10 minutes
Below shoulders	15 minutes

6.2 Shampooing hair

It is essential to cleanse the hair and scalp to remove dirt, oil and any product build up that may act as a barrier to future services. This section covers the shampoo technique and the types of products that are used. The stylist will choose which products must be used. If you have not been told, you should ask. Using the incorrect product will have a negative effect on the hair.

pH, acidity and alkalinity

The pH of a product is measured on a scale of 0–14. Water has a pH of 7 and is said to be neutral. Products with a pH of less than 7 are described as acid and they close the cuticle. Products with a pH of more than 7 are described as alkaline and they open the cuticle. Shampoos and conditioners are usually 5.5–6 on the pH scale.

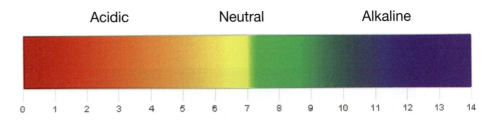

Figure 6.12 pH colour scale

Shampooing products

Choice of shampoo is determined by:

* type, texture and condition of the hair and scalp
* purpose of the shampoo
* treatment after the shampoo.

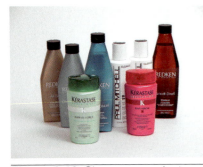

Figure 6.13 Shampoo products

Types of shampoos and ingredients

There are many types of shampoo that are used for different hair or scalp types. The table below shows the ingredients that may be contained in the relevant shampoo.

Table 5.2 Types of shampoo and their ingredients

Type	Ingredients
Normal hair	Rosemary Soya
Dry/damaged hair	Almond oil Coconut Lanolin
Oily hair	Lemon Egg white
Dandruff	Coal tar Zinc pyrithione Selenium sulphide

Online activity 6.3   **www**

Scrambled words

Purpose of shampoo

The purpose of shampoo is to:

- cleanse the hair
- remove any products
- prepare the hair for the next service.

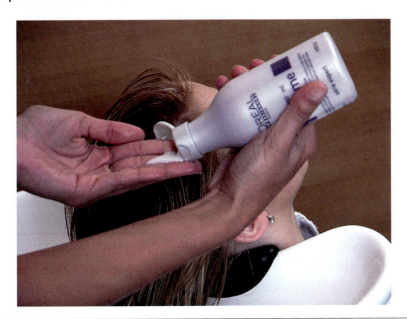

Figure 6.14 Dispensing shampoo

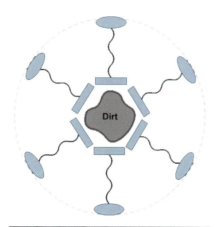

Figure 6.15 Shampoo molecules surrounding the dirt

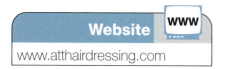

Definition

Emulsify: To blend two liquids that wouldn't naturally combine together.

Website www

www.atthairdressing.com

Definitions

Vigorously: Active strength.

Seborrhoea: A condition in which excess sebum is produced from the sebaceous gland.

How shampoos work – shampoo and its relationship with water

The detergent molecules of the shampoo have a head and a tail. The head is hydrophilic, which means it attracts water and the tail is hydrophobic, which means it repels water. The hydrophobic end of the molecule is attracted to dirt on the hair. It surrounds the dirt and suspends it in the water. This action is aided by agitation from the massage.

When the hair is rinsed, the hydrophilic heads pull the dirt or oil from the hair and carry it away with the flow of water. The detergent during the shampooing process acts as an emulsifying agent because it holds the oil and water together.

Massage techniques

The following techniques for massaging are used when shampooing hair (see online video):

- effleurage and
- rotary.

Effleurage massage is a gentle, smooth, stroking movement using the palms of the hands. It is used more on long, dense hair to avoid tangling and ensure thorough cleaning. Rotary massage uses the pads of the fingers in quick, circular movements.

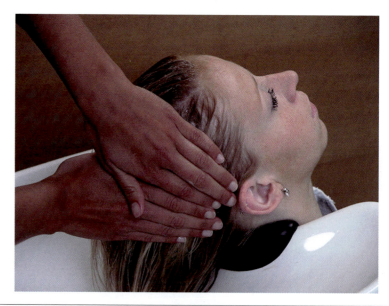

Figure 6.16 Be careful when massaging

Client care

Some clients are more sensitive to pressure than others. When massaging, be aware of the client's tolerance levels. Look for warning signs that you may be massaging too vigorously. Do not over-stimulate the scalp if the client suffers from seborrhoea, dizziness or high blood pressure.

Online activity 6.4   WWW

Round the board

Shampooing procedure

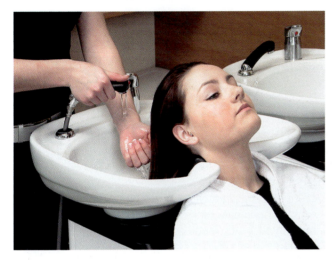

Figure 6.17 After the client has been gowned correctly and is sitting comfortably at the washbasin the temperature of the water should be tested on the inside of the shampooist's wrist. This is to prevent scalding the client.

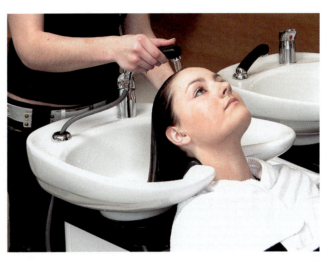

Figure 6.18 Check the temperature with the client, which may vary. Some clients may require the water cooler or warmer. Apply water to hair.

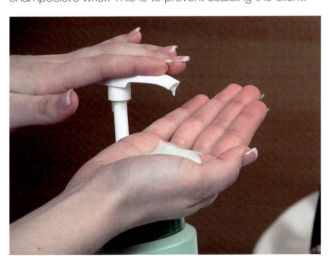

Figure 6.19 Dispense the shampoo into the palm of the hand then gently rub both hands together to evenly distribute the shampoo through the hair. Shampoo that is applied to one area of the scalp is difficult to distribute evenly. Use the amount of shampoo recommended by the manufacturer. Do not use more than the recommended amount.

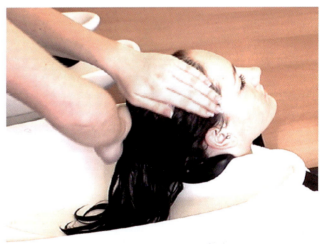

Figure 6.20 The shampoo is applied using effleurage massage (online video).

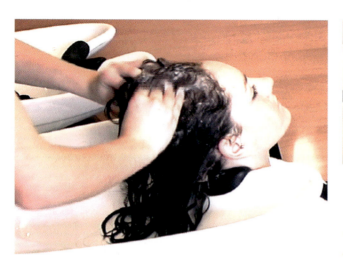

Figure 6.21 The second massage movement used during shampooing is rotary. Begin at the front hairline and work towards the ears. Repeat this action several times. Pay particular attention to the hairline of female client's as this is where residuals of make-up and face creams are found.

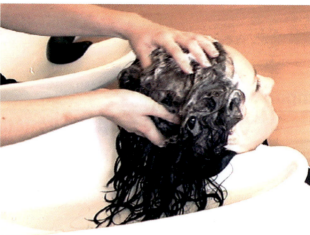

Figure 6.22 Then move the fingers from the front hairline over the crown and down towards the nape. Next move the hands over the sides of the head continuing the massage movement. Repeat this formation several times. Make sure that the scalp area is covered thoroughly. Pay attention to the nape area, particularly when shampooing at a backwash basin. It may be necessary to repeat this process to remove a build up of products.

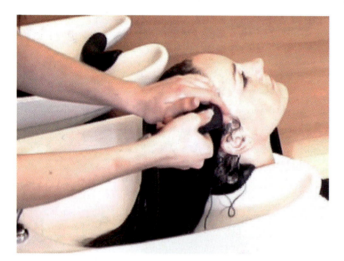

Figure 6.23 Rinse the hair thoroughly, so that it is completely free of shampoo. Start rinsing from the front hairline if using a backwash or the nape of the neck if using a forward basin and work through the rest of the hair. Remove excess moisture with a towel and comb through.

Online activity 6.5

Drag into correct order

6.3 Applying conditioners to the hair

Conditioners will improve the condition of the hair and allow it to be controlled effectively. The stylist will have chosen which products and tools must be used and if you have not been told, you should ask. Using the wrong product will have a negative effect on the hair.

Types of conditioner

Conditioners work by closing the hair cuticle. This makes it easier to comb the hair through. The types of conditioner are:

- surface conditioners
- treatment conditioners.

Surface conditioners

These work on the surface layer of the hair, coating the hair shaft and filling in any gaps in the cuticle layer that have been caused by previous treatments.

Treatment conditioners

These conditioners penetrate the cuticle and help to repair damage by adding protein. As these conditioners add protein to the hair they are known as substantive products and will strengthen the hair structure.

Safety first

Using the wrong product will have a negative effect on the hair, so always ask the stylist before you shampoo.

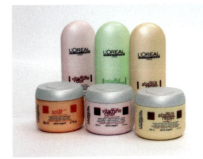

Figure 6.24 Conditioners

 Definitions

Hair shaft: The part of the hair that is above the skin.

Cuticle: Outer layer of the hair shaft.

Protein: Hair structure, made from amino acids.

Substantive: Having weight or value. An important product.

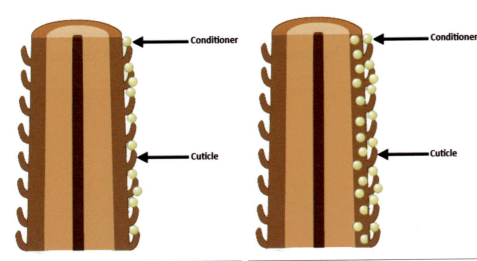

Figure 6.25 Surface conditioner   **Figure 6.26** Treatment conditioner

Tools and equipment

Heat can complement the conditioning process. Always read the manufacturers' instructions before using added heat. Heat can be added using a hood dryer, accelerator or steamer.

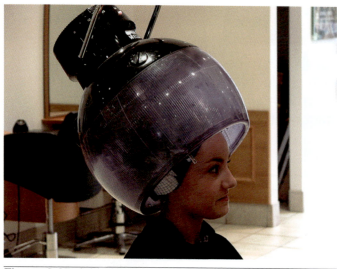

Figure 6.27 Added heat

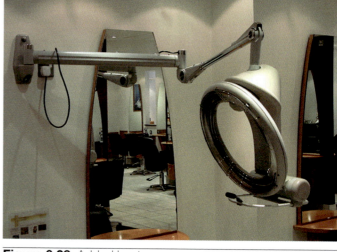

Figure 6.28 Added heat

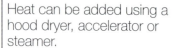

Massage techniques

The following techniques are used for massaging when conditioning hair:

- effleurage
- petrissage.

Effleurage massage is a gentle, smooth, stroking movement using the palms of the hands. It is used more on long, dense hair to avoid tangling and ensure thorough cleaning.

Petrissage massage movements are performed using the pads of the fingers in slow circular, kneading movements around the hairline and over the scalp. It is a firm massage, which improves circulation, relaxes the client and helps to break down any fatty adhesions to the scalp. If the hair is sparse, be very careful to avoid 'pulling' it.

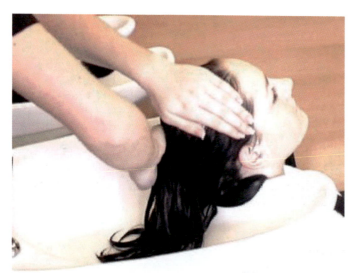

Figure 6.29 Effleurage massage

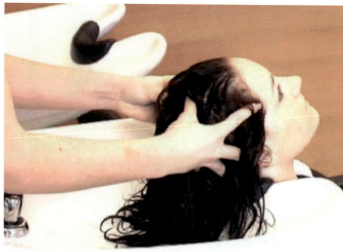

Figure 6.30 Petrissage massage

Online activity 6.6 **WWW**

Five in a row

Application of conditioners

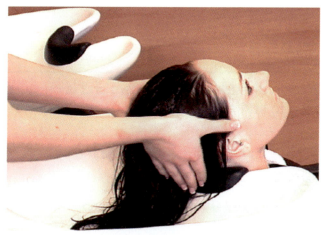

Figure 6.31 Most conditioners are applied at the basin after the hair has been shampooed and towel dried. The product is evenly distributed through the hair using the effleurage massage technique.

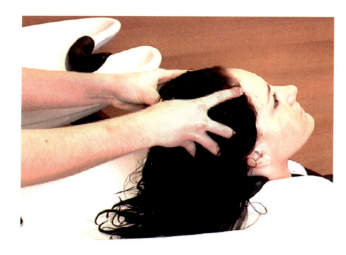

Figure 6.32 The product is then massaged through the hair and into the scalp using the petrissage technique.

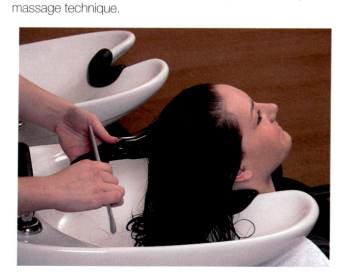

Figure 6.33 Comb through from ends to roots.

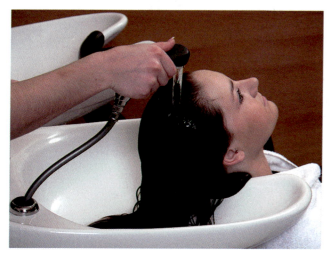

Figure 6.34 Surface conditioners are rinsed off straight away. Treatment conditioners are left in the hair for the recommended time, which is approximately 5–10 minutes. Ensure all product has been rinsed out. Remove any excess moisture and comb the hair.

Now complete all the worksheets in the following section.

WORKSHEETS

6.4 Worksheets

You can carry out these worksheets during your study of a chapter or unit, or at the end. If your college or training company is registered with ATT Training, lots more of these worksheets are available. Write your answers directly in the book – but only if you own it of course – if it is a library or college book, use a separate piece of paper!

Dermatitis

This is a very common skin disease in hairdressers and is caused by hands being exposed to certain products and carrying out wet-work regularly.

Dermatitis can be prevented by taking a number of precautions.

Note down what these precautions are:

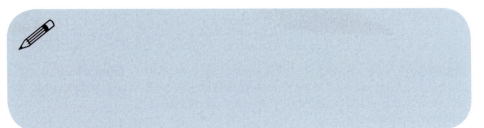

How shampoos work

Shampoo and its relationship with water:

The detergent molecules of the shampoo have a head and tail. The head is hydrophilic which means it attracts water and the tail is hydrophobic which means it repels water.

Label this diagram:

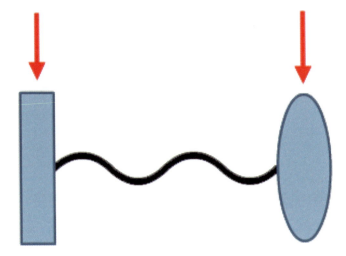

Figure 6.35 Shampoo molecule

The hydrophobic end of the molecule is attracted to the dirt on the hair. It surrounds the dirt and suspends it in the water. This action is aided by agitation from the massage.

Complete the diagram below to illustrate this:

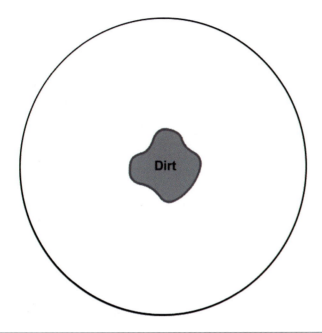

Figure 6.36 Dirt

When the hair is rinsed, the hydrophilic head pulls the dirt or oil from the hair and carries it away with the flow of the water. During the shampooing process, the detergent acts as an emulsifying agent because it holds the oil and water together.

Types of conditioner

Surface conditioners work on the surface layer of the hair. They coat the hair shaft . . .

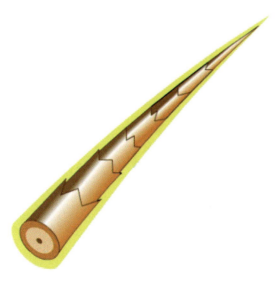

Figure 6.37 Surface conditioners coat the hair shaft

. . . and fill in any gaps in the cuticle layer that have been caused by previous treatments.

Label this diagram

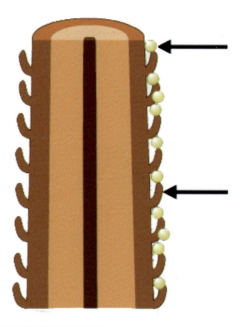

Figure 6.38 Surface conditioner

Treatment conditioners penetrate the cuticle and help to repair damage by adding protein. They are known as substantive products and strengthen the hair structure.

Label this diagram

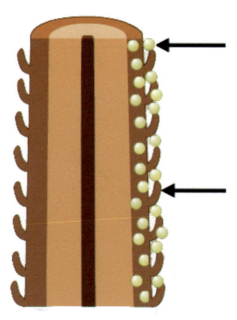

Figure 6.39 Treatment conditioner

6.5 Assessment

Well done! If you have studied all the content of this unit you may be ready to test your knowledge.

Check out the 'Preparing for assessments' section in Chapter 1 if you have not already done so. Always remember:

- You can only do your best if you have . . .
  - studied hard
  - completed the activities
  - completed the worksheets
  - practised, practised, practised
  - and then revised!

Now carry out the online multiple-choice quiz

. . . and good luck in the final exam, which will be arranged by your tutor/ assessor.

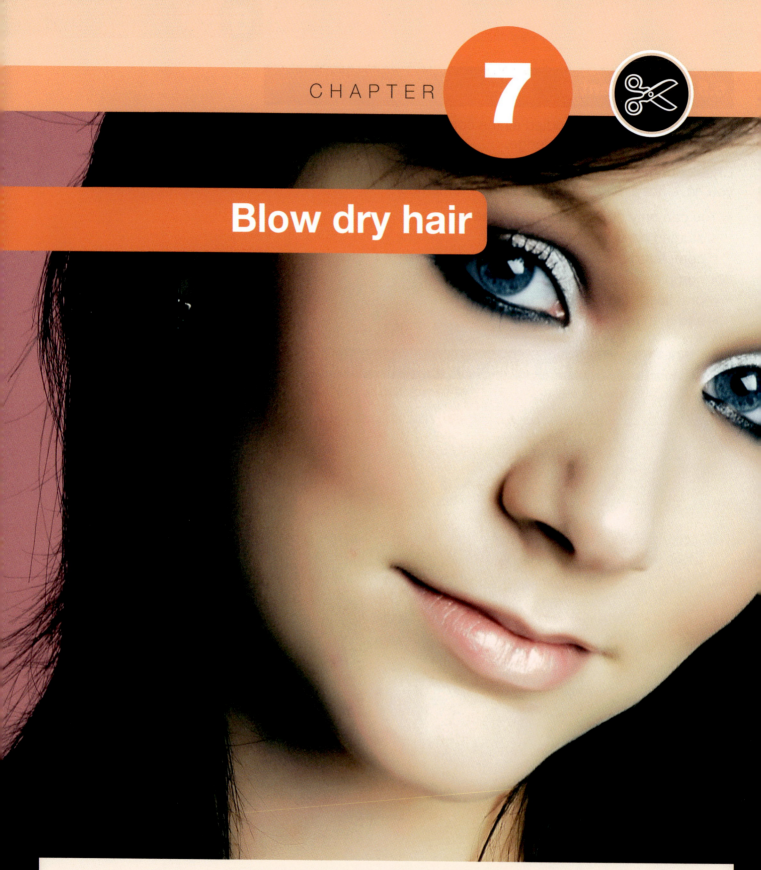

Blow dry hair

This chapter covers the NVQ/SVQ unit GH2, Blow dry hair

This styling technique is a crucial part of the hairdressing service that your salon offers its clients. You will be carrying out basic blow drying methods, always following the stylist's instructions.

In this chapter you will learn about:

■ maintaining effective and safe methods of working when drying hair

■ blow drying hair.

CHAPTER 7 BLOW DRY HAIR: CONTENTS, SCREENS AND ACTIVITIES

Key:

Sections from the book are set in this colour
Screens available online are set in this colour
Online activity screens are set in this colour

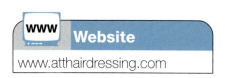

Working safely

Introduction
Safe methods of working when blow drying hair
Hair is hygroscopic
Products used during blow drying
Select correct boxes
Blow drying tools and equipment
Brushes

Hand dryers
Comfort during blow drying 1
Round the board
Comfort during blow drying 2
Keep work area tidy
Suggested service times

Blow dry hair

Introduction
Applying products
Mousse
Serum
Lotion
Cream
Gels
Hairspray
Five in a row
Controlling styling tools
Blow drying hair to create volume

Blow drying hair into shape
Round the board
Blow drying hair to create movement
Blow drying long hair straight 1
Blow drying long hair straight 2
Correct selection
Worksheet – Hair is hygroscopic
Worksheet – Blow drying tools and equipment
Worksheet – Blow drying hair to create movement
Online multiple choice quiz

Safety first

Chapter 2 covers health and safety working methods in more detail. Refer to this unit if needed.

Definitions

Alpha keratin: Hair in its natural unstretched state.

Beta keratin: The stretched (wet) state of hair.

7.1 Working safely

This section covers the health and safety knowledge with regards to techniques, products and equipment used during blow drying.

Hair is hygroscopic

This means that it has the ability to absorb moisture.

Wet hair can be stretched nearly double its normal length. This is called elasticity. Wet hair in its stretched state is called the 'beta keratin'. When it is in the natural state (unstretched), the hair is called the 'alpha keratin'. The reason hair stretches is because the hydrogen bonds are broken down by water. These properties allow us to alter the shape of hair. When heat is applied, the hydrogen bonds can be re-formed into a new shape. The humidity in the air affects the structure of the hair by making it feel damp. This will take the hair back to its natural state.

WWW

View the online video to learn more about the hair in its various states

Products used during styling and finishing

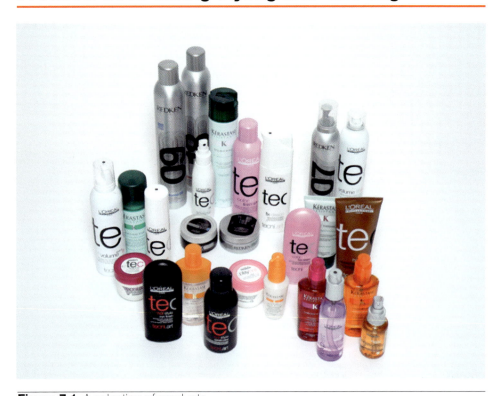

Figure 7.1 A selection of products

These include:

- mousse
- serum
- lotion
- cream
- gel
- heat protector
- spray.

To prevent product wastage, only use the amount needed according to manufacturers' instructions.

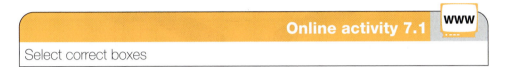

Online activity 7.1 **www**

Select correct boxes

Blow drying tools and equipment

Tools and equipment used for blow drying hair include brushes and hand dryers. Keep tools and equipment clean and sterilised at all times to prevent product building up and causing sticky areas. As the tools and equipment are used, the hair may become attached to these areas and become damaged.

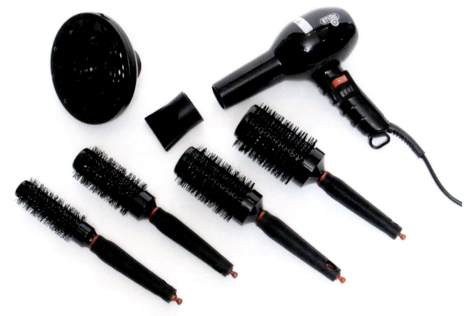

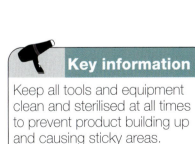

Key information

Keep all tools and equipment clean and sterilised at all times to prevent product building up and causing sticky areas.

Figure 7.2 Range of blow drying equipment

Brushes

It is essential to have different-sized circular brushes so that you can produce appropriate sized curls according to the client's wishes. Large circular brushes are used for longer hair. Flat brushes are used to straighten hair.

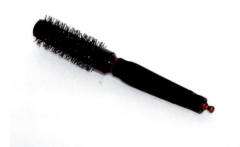

Figure 7.3 Small circular brush

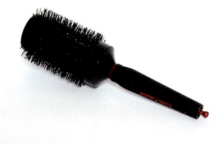

Figure 7.4 Large circular brush

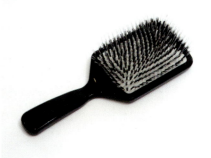

Figure 7.5 Flat brush

Hand dryers

There are many different types of hand dryer. You should be able to change the temperature and speed. The dryer will be used for long periods of time, so should be able to handle this. The hand dryer should also be easy to use and lightweight.

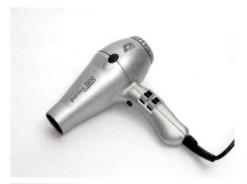

Figure 7.6 Hand dryer

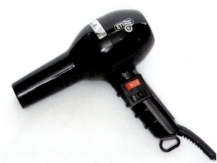

Figure 7.7 Hand dryer

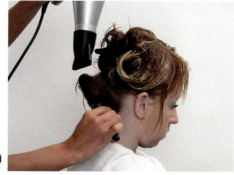

Figure 7.8 Hand dryer in use

Comfort during blow drying

When the client arrives for a blow dry, they will probably already be wearing a gown to protect their clothes. If the client has just had their hair shampooed and has a towel wrapped around their hair, you should ensure that water does not drip on their clothes when you remove the towel. Using the towel, gently remove any excess moisture from the hair and then carefully place a clean dry towel around their shoulders before the blow dry.

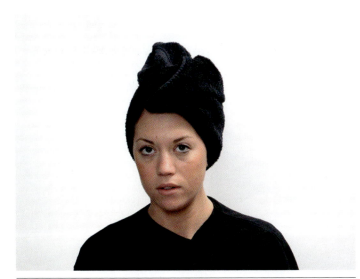

Figure 7.9 Client after their shampoo

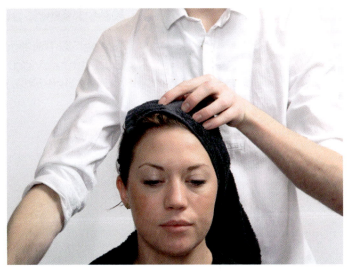

Figure 7.10 Removing the towel carefully

Online activity 7.2 www

Round the board

Whilst blow drying the client's hair, it is important for you to move around your client's head. However, the client's comfort should be considered at all times. Their back should be positioned right to the back of the chair and as flat as possible. They should have both feet on the footrest or the floor. Not only will this be a more comfortable position for the client, but it also enables you to create a balanced hairstyle.

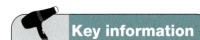

Key information

If the client has just had their hair shampooed and has a towel wrapped around their hair, you should ensure that water does not drip on their clothes when you remove the towel.

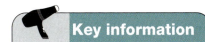

Key information

Your own comfort should be considered. Check your posture is correct, ensuring that your client's seat is at the correct height for you to work.

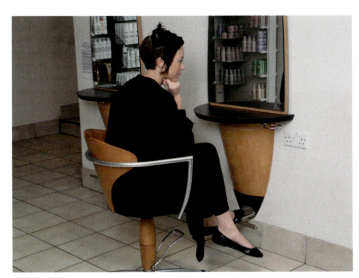

Figure 7.11 Incorrect posture

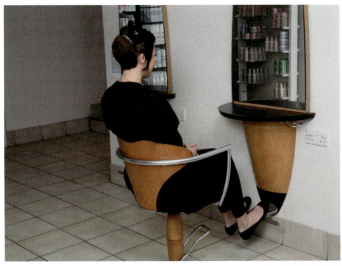

Figure 7.12 Correct posture

Keep work area tidy

Gather all the equipment and products you will need before you start the service. Ensure that your work area is tidy and free from clutter. See Chapter 5 for more information on cleaning in the salon.

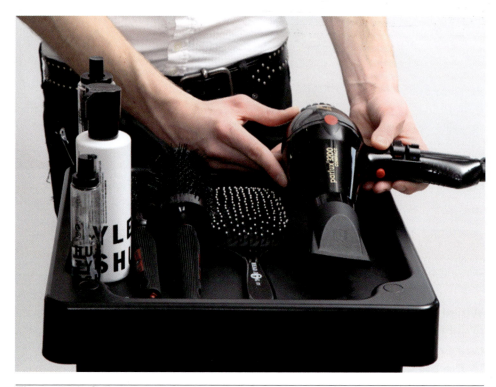

Figure 7.13 Gather up your equipment and products needed for blow drying

Suggested service times

Viable times for blow drying are as follows:

Table 7.1 Service times

Length of hair	Time
Above shoulders	30 minutes
Below shoulders	45 minutes

7.2 Blow drying hair

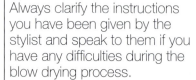

Key information

Always clarify the instructions you have been given by the stylist and speak to them if you have any difficulties during the blow drying process.

Before blow drying the client's hair you will be given instructions by the stylist. Ensure that you follow these carefully. They may wish for you to section and dry the hair in a particular order, so that is what you must do. Always clarify the instructions you have been given. Always speak to the stylist if you have any difficulties during blow drying. Check that the client is comfortable throughout the blow drying process.

Applying products

Before blow drying, you may be asked to apply styling products to the client's hair. Only use products on the client's hair if the stylist has asked you to.

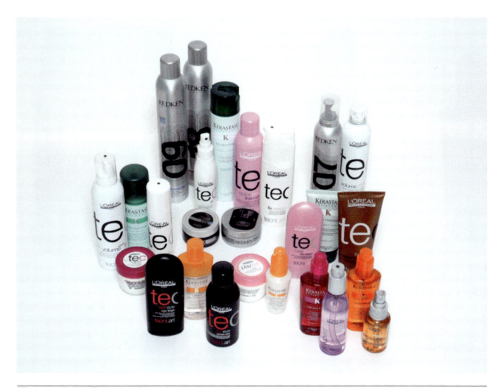

Figure 7.14 Range of products

Mousse

Mousse is available in different strengths. It is applied to wet hair with the hands and will hold style in place and achieve a soft effect.

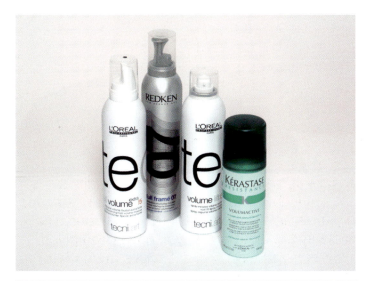

Figure 7.15 A range of mousse products

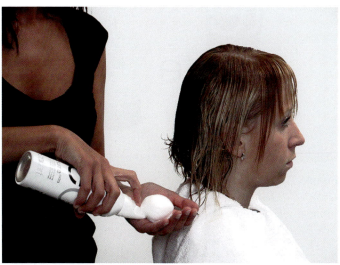

Figure 7.16 Mousse is applied to wet hair

Serum

Hair serum makes hair look shiny and in better condition. This product must be used sparingly as it is very concentrated. It can make hair appear lank or greasy.

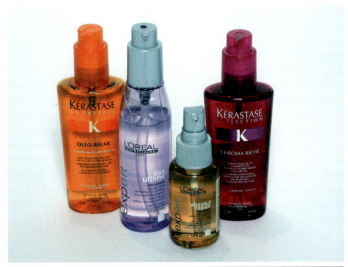

Figure 7.17 A range of serums

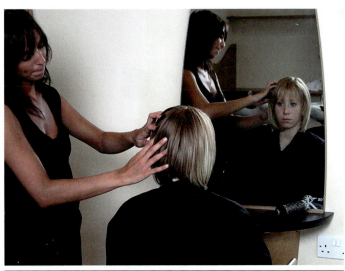

Figure 7.18 Use sparingly!

Lotion

Lotions are used on wet hair and are produced as a light cream or liquid. They help to maintain the style for longer.

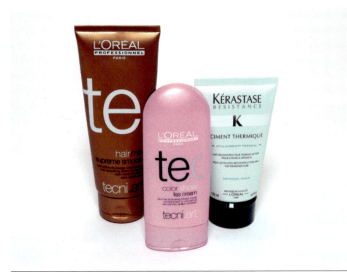

Figure 7.19 Different types of lotion

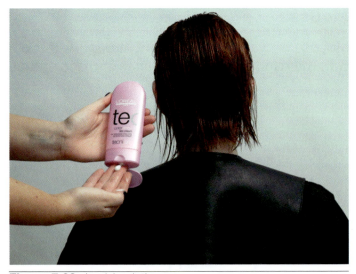

Figure 7.20 Applying lotion

Cream

Creams can be used on either wet or dry hair and should be used sparingly. They are used to moisturise the hair and add curl definition.

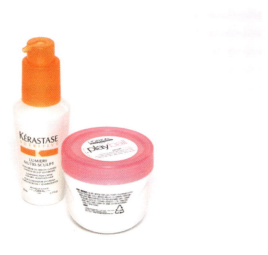

Figure 7.21 Creams

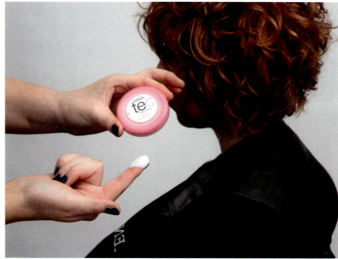

Figure 7.22 Applying cream

Gel

Gels are designed to be used on either wet or dry hair. They complement and give definition to the style.

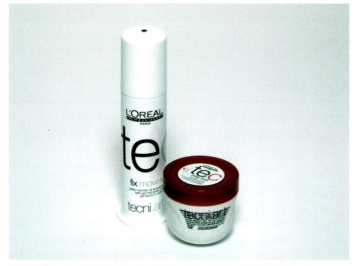

Figure 7.23 Gels

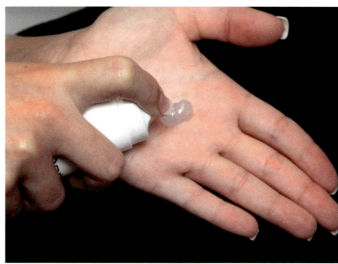

Figure 7.24 Applying gel

7

Hairspray

Hairspray holds the hair in place and protects the hair from the weather and humidity. It comes in different strengths and, as most hairsprays are water soluble, it is easily removed from the hair by brushing or wetting. When applying hairspray, the spray should be pointed away from the client's face. This can be achieved by standing in front of your client when you are applying the product. It should be held approximately 10–12 inches from the head.

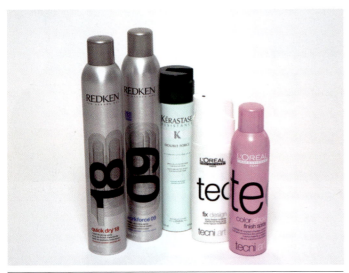

Figure 7.25 Hairspray

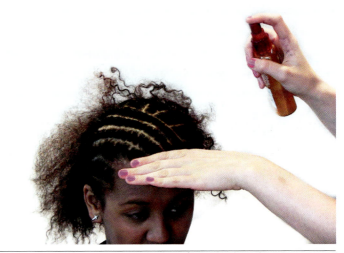

Figure 7.26 Spray 10–12 inches from the head

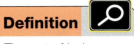

www   **Online activity 7.3**

Five in a row

Controlling styling tools

When using any brush, it is important to be gentle otherwise the hair can become tangled or damaged. This is also uncomfortable for the client. An even tension should be kept at all times to avoid overstretching the hair. When drying, the angle of the brush determines how much root movement (lift or bounce) is achieved. Long hair will not allow much root lift because of the length and weight of the hair.

Definition

Tension: The act of being stretched.

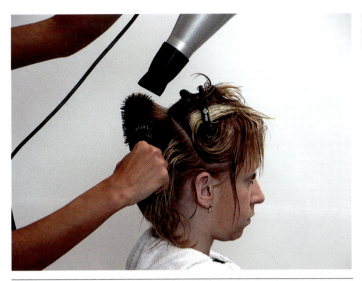

Figure 7.27 *Control your styling tools*

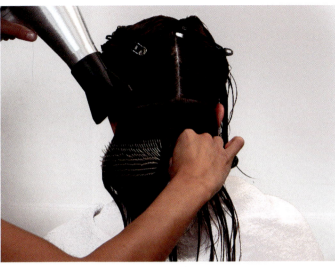

Figure 7.28 *Long hair will not allow much root lift*

Blow drying hair to create volume

(See online video)

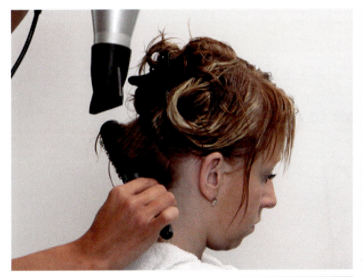

Figure 7.29 Starting at the nape area, dry the hair by curling around the brush. Use a small, medium or large circular brush for the required curl strength. When drying curly or long hair into shape on a client, the position of the head is very important. When working at the nape area, the head has to be angled forward for efficient operation

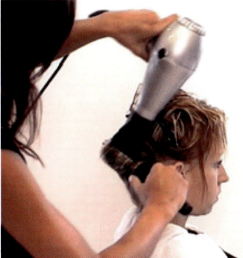

Figure 7.30 When placing the hand dryer over the hair, keep the nozzle of the hand dryer moving to prevent the hair and scalp being burnt. The direction of the air flow from the hand dryer must be directed along the hair shaft from roots to ends and in the same direction as the brush strokes. This will ensure an even and smoother finish

www **Website**

www.atthairdressing.com

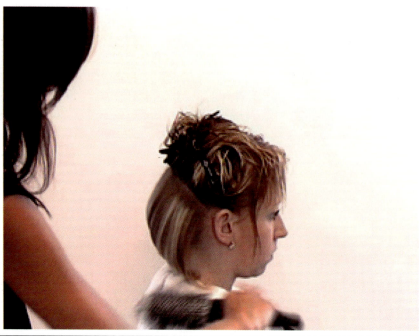

Figure 7.31 Work methodically through each section ensuring root lift and smoothness of curl formation until the hair is dry

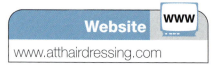
Website **www**
www.atthairdressing.com

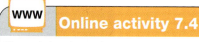
www **Online activity 7.4**
Round the board

Blow drying hair to create movement

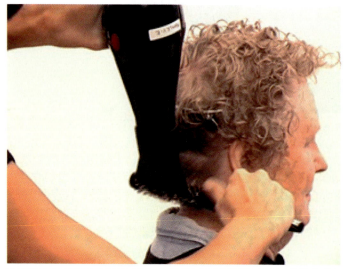

Figure 7.32 Section the hair after application of product. Starting at the nape area, dry the hair by curling the hair around the brush. Use a small, medium or large spiral brush for the required curl strength (online video)

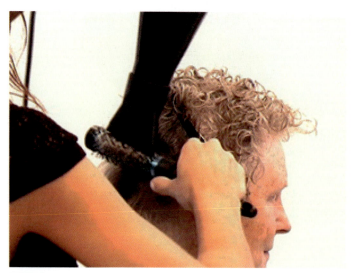

Figure 7.33 Work methodically through each section (online video)

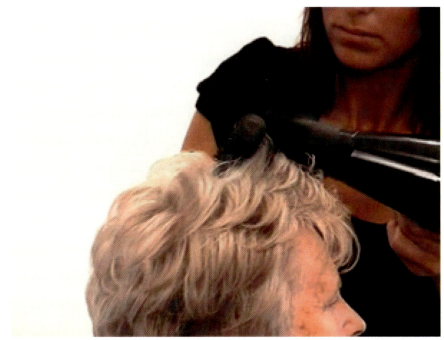

Figure 7.34 Ensure root lift and smoothness of curl formation until the hair is dry (online video)

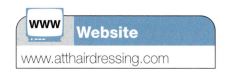

www Website
www.atthairdressing.com

Blow drying long hair straight

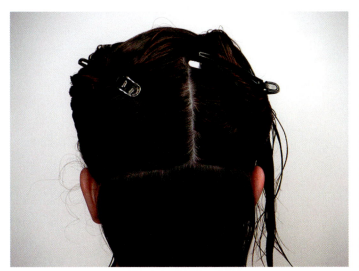

Figure 7.35 After applying suitable product, section the hair and secure the hair not to be dried at this time with clips

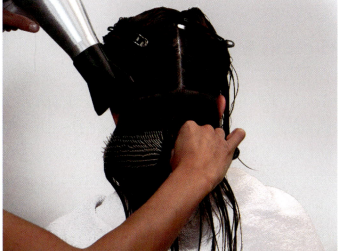

Figure 7.36 To achieve a smooth effect a flat or a very large circular brush can be used. Create neat sections and dry the hair from roots to end ensuring each section is thoroughly dry before going on to the next section

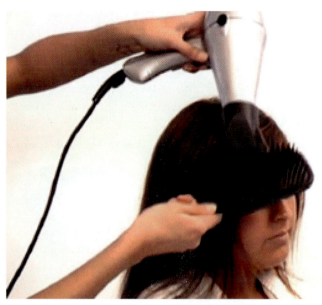

Figure 7.37 As the hairdresser works up the head in sections, the head will need to be altered to a more upright position. This will assist the hairdresser

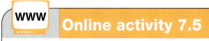

WWW   Online activity 7.5

Round the board

Now complete all the worksheets in the following section.

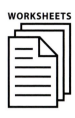

7.3 Worksheets

You can carry out these worksheets during your study of a chapter or unit, or at the end. If your college or training company is registered with ATT Training, lots more of these worksheets are available. Write your answers directly in the book – but only if you own it of course – if it is a library or college book, use a separate piece of paper!

Hair is hygroscopic

Hair is hygroscopic. This means that it has the ability to absorb moisture. Wet hair can be stretched to nearly double its normal length. This is called elasticity. Wet hair in its stretched state is called 'beta keratin'. When it is in the natural state (unstretched), the hair is called 'alpha keratin'. The reason why hair stretches is because the hydrogen bonds are broken down by water. These properties allow us to alter the shape of the hair. When heat is applied, the hydrogen bonds can be re-formed into a new shape. Humidity in the air will affect the structure of the hair by making it feel damp. This will take the hair back to its natural state.

State five treatments carried out in your salon that involve the above process.

1.

2.

3.

4.

5.

Blow drying tools and equipment

Keep all tools and equipment clean and sterilised at all times to prevent product building up and causing sticky areas. As the tools and equipment are used, the hair may become attached to these areas and become damaged.

Name the different tools and equipment that you think are used during blow drying. Suggest why you think that each might be used:

Product	Use

Blow drying hair to create movement

Fill in the missing words. Refer to the previous chapter or the online learning screens for assistance.

Section the hair after application of _____.

Starting at the nape area, dry the hair by curling the hair around the _____. Use a small, medium or large spiral brush for the required curl strength.

Work methodically through each _____ ensuring root lift and smoothness of curl formation until the hair is dry.

7.4 Assessment

Well done! If you have studied all the content of this unit you may be ready to test your knowledge.

Check out the 'Preparing for assessments' section in Chapter 1 if you have not already done so, and always remember:

- You can only do your best if you have . . .
  - ○ studied hard
  - ○ completed the activities
  - ○ completed the worksheets
  - ○ practised, practised, practised
  - ○ and then revised!

 Now carry out the online multiple-choice quiz

. . . and good luck in the final exam, which will be arranged by your tutor/ assessor.

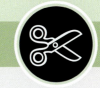
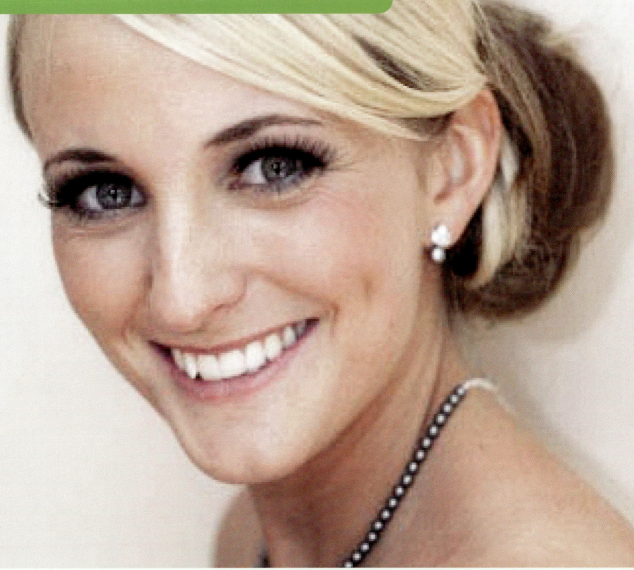

Assist with hair colouring services

This chapter covers the NVQ/SVQ unit GH4, Assist with hair colouring services

There are many methods and techniques when colouring hair. At this level you will be helping the stylist and following their instructions at all times.

In this chapter you will learn about:

- maintaining effective and safe methods of working when assisting with the colouring service

- removing colouring and lightening products.

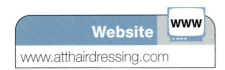

CHAPTER 8 ASSIST WITH COLOURING AND LIGHTENING SERVICES: CONTENTS, SCREENS AND ACTIVITIES

Key:
Sections from the book are set in this colour
Screens available online are set in this colour
Online activity screens are set in this colour

Working safely

Introduction

Safe methods of working when assisting with colouring services

Client preparation and comfort

Personal protective equipment (PPE)

COSHH

Posture and deportment

Keeping the work area clean and tidy and checking levels of products

Five in a row

Remove colouring and lightening products

Introduction

Test water before and during rinsing

Removal of quasi-permanent, permanent and lighteners 1

Removal of quasi-permanent, permanent and lighteners 2

Removal of quasi-permanent, permanent and lighteners 3

Drag into correct order

Removal of semi-permanent colour

Removing foils and packets

Problems during colour rinsing

After the rinsing process

Round the board

Worksheet – Posture and deportment

Worksheet – Removal of colour

Worksheet – Problems during colour rinsing

Online multiple choice quiz

8.1 Working safely

Working with colours and lighteners means that you will be working with chemicals. Therefore you must be very careful to protect the client and yourself from these chemicals at all times. Chapter 2 covers health and safety working methods in more detail. Refer to this unit if needed.

Client preparation and comfort

Ensure that your client's clothing is protected during the service. As you will be rinsing off colour and/or lighteners, the client should be prepared using a plastic cape in addition to gown and towel. Client comfort should be considered at all times. Ensure that the client's neck is supported. See Chapter 6 for more information.

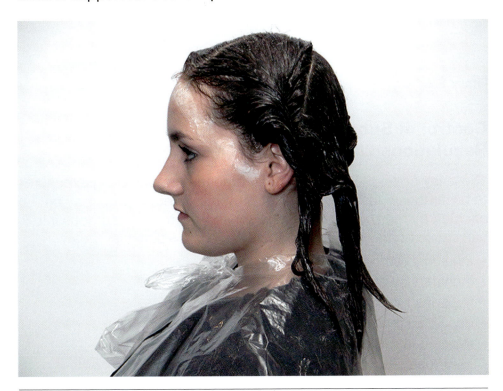

Figure 8.1 Ensure client's clothing is protected

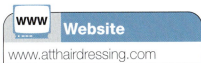

www **Website**

www.atthairdressing.com

Personal protective equipment (PPE)

When removing colouring products from the client's hair, ensure that you are wearing the correct PPE at all times. Colouring products contain chemicals and so will be hazardous to your health. This will avoid you developing contact dermatitis. See Chapter 2 for more information.

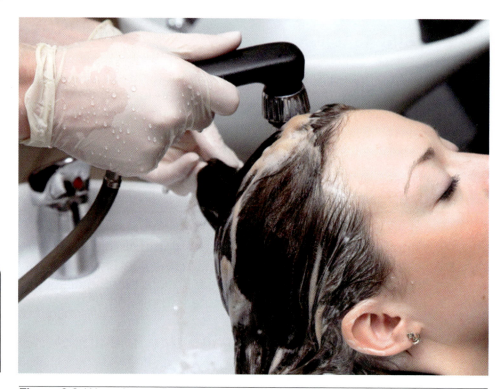

Figure 8.2 Wear gloves when you are removing colouring products from the hair

Control of Substances Hazardous to Health Regulations 2002 (COSHH)

These lay down the essential requirements for controlling exposure to hazardous substances and for protecting people who may be affected by them. A substance is considered to be hazardous if it can cause harm to the body. It only poses a risk if it is:

- inhaled (breathed in)
- ingested (swallowed)
- in contact with the skin
- absorbed through the skin
- injected into the body
- introduced into the body via cuts etc.

For more information about the COSHH regulations, refer to Chapter 2.

Posture and deportment

Make sure you check your posture when you are at the washbasin to avoid injury. The back should be kept straight, bend from the knees, feet apart with weight evenly distributed. If the spine is bent the back will have excess strain and the body will tire. The lungs will also be constricted; this lowers the intake of oxygen, which induces tiredness.

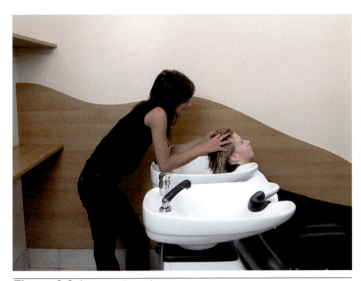

Figure 8.3 Incorrect posture

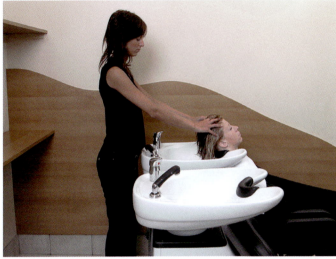

Figure 8.4 Correct posture

Keeping the work area clean and tidy and checking levels of products

Your work area should always be kept clean and tidy. Colouring equipment and waste materials including foils and meshes must be removed from the sink and surrounding areas. Dispose of them according to your salon policy.

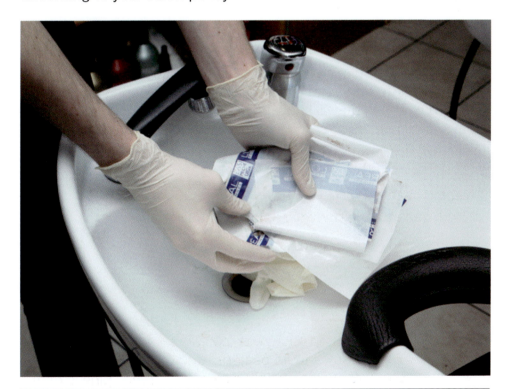

Figure 8.5 Remove waste materials from the sink

Ensure that colouring bowls are washed out as soon as the stylist is finished. Dilute with water before emptying down the sink.

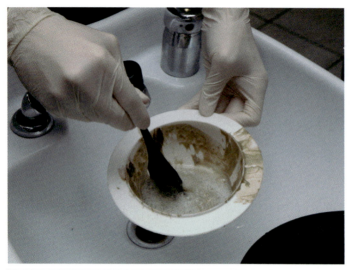

Figure 8.6 Dilute colouring bowls with water and empty down the sink

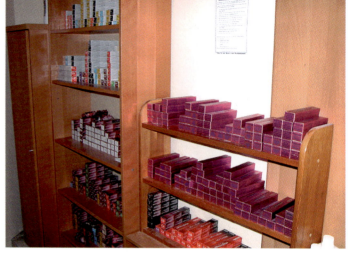

Figure 8.7 Check stock of colouring products

Key information

Chapter 5 covers stock levels, cleanliness and tidy work practices in more detail. Refer to this unit if needed.

Check levels of colouring products to maintain stock requirements.

www **Online activity 8.1**

Five in a row

8.2 Removing colouring and lightening products

Safety first ⚠

You must always take care, as after the hair has been coloured and lightened it will be in a weakened state.

Before removing colour and/or lightening products from the hair, it is important to understand which method of colouring has been carried out. Then you will know how to remove the colour. You must always take care, as after the hair has been coloured and lightened it will be in a weakened state. Always check with the stylist, the correct method and order for removal.

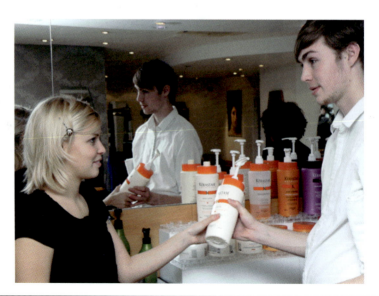

Figure 8.8 Ask the stylist for the correct method

Test water before and during rinsing

After the client has been gowned correctly and is sitting at the washbasin comfortably the temperature of the water should be tested on the inside of your wrist. This is to prevent scalding the client. Check the temperature with the client, which may vary. Some clients may require the water cooler or warmer.

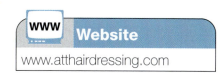

Website

www.atthairdressing.com

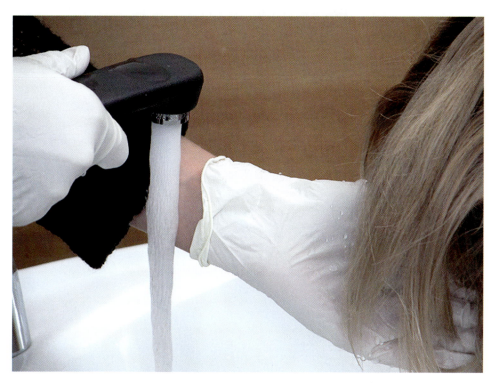

Figure 8.9 Test the water on your wrist before rinsing

Removal of quasi-permanent, permanent and lightening product

When rinsing a full head of permanent colour it is important to emulsify the hairline. This will make it easier to remove the colour from the skin. To do this, massage the area using your fingertips. An emulsion will then be formed which can then be rinsed away. Rinse the hair starting with the forehead, then move on to the sides of the head and finally through the lengths.

 Definition

Emulsify: To blend two liquids that wouldn't naturally combine together.

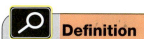

The associated learning screen shows a video of emulsifying the hairline

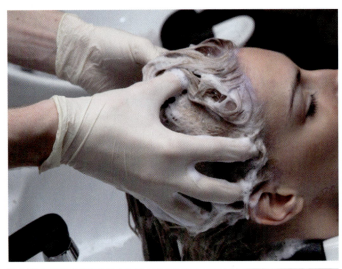

Figure 8.10 Dispense the shampoo into the palm of the hand, then gently rub both hands together to evenly distribute the shampoo through the hair. Apply to the hair. Use the amount of shampoo recommended by the manufacturer. Do not use more than the recommended amount

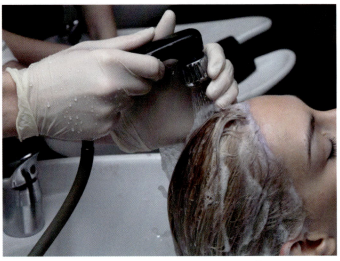

Figure 8.11 Massage the shampoo into the head and once the whole area is covered, rinse. The water temperature and pressure must be tested with the client

Key information

If the stylist has asked for two washes then repeat this procedure.

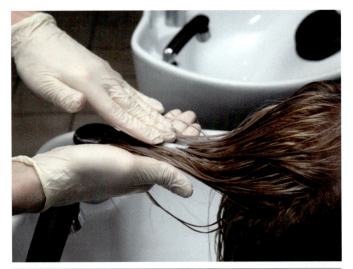

Figure 8.12 Condition the hair with a suitable conditioner as instructed by the stylist

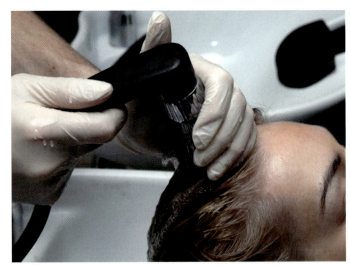

Figure 8.13 Rinse off

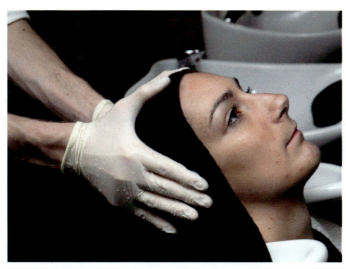

Figure 8.14 Remove excess moisture with a gentle towel-through

Online activity 8.2 **www**

Drag into correct order

Removal of semi-permanent colour

Semi-permanent colour can just be rinsed away. There is no need to condition as the colouring products have conditioning properties within them.

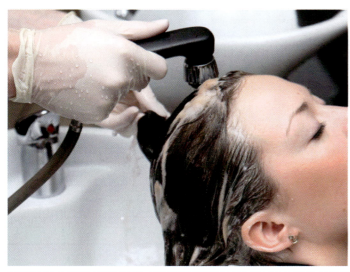

Figure 8.15 To remove semi-permanent colour, rinse . . .

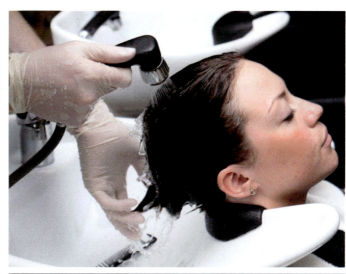

Figure 8.16 . . . until the water runs clear

Removing foils and packets

Foils and packets must be carefully unfolded before removal. Product should be rinsed from each individual one.

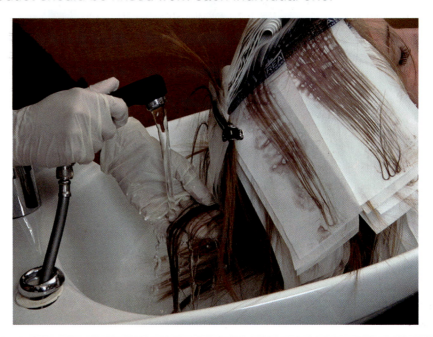

Figure 8.17 Remove packets carefully

Problems during colour rinsing

Table 8.1 shows you the problems that can occur during the rinsing process and what action you should take to resolve them. Study it carefully.

Table 8.1 Colour rinsing problems

Problem	Action
Colour from foils or highlights is leaking onto the other parts of the hair	Ask stylist for help
Colour has gone into client's eye	Ask the client to hold cotton wool that has been dampened with water to their eye
	Ask stylist or other senior member of staff for help
Colour still on hair after rinsing	Re-shampoo and condition
Client's skin has colour on	Use stain remover as soon as possible
Colour has gone onto the client's gown	Give the client a fresh gown or remove the colour through sponging

After the rinsing process

When you have finished the rinsing process, shampooed and conditioned, ask the client to sit upright. Remove the client's towel from around their shoulders and wrap around the hair. Help the client to the workstation and inform the stylist that the client is now ready for them.

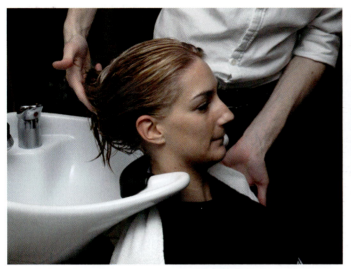

Figure 8.18 Assisting the client to an upright position

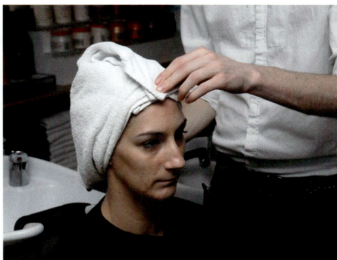

Figure 8.19 Wrapping a towel around the hair

Online activity 8.3   `WWW`

Round the board

Now complete all of the worksheets in the following section.

WORKSHEETS

8.3 Worksheets

You can carry out these worksheets during your study of a chapter or unit, or at the end. If your college or training company is registered with ATT Training, lots more of these worksheets are available. Write your answers directly in the book – but only if you own it of course – if it is a library or college book, use a separate piece of paper!

Posture and deportment

Make sure you check your posture when you are at the washbasin to avoid injury.

Indicate which of these photos shows the correct way to stand:

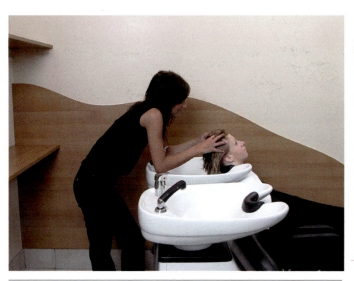

Figure 8.20 Posture

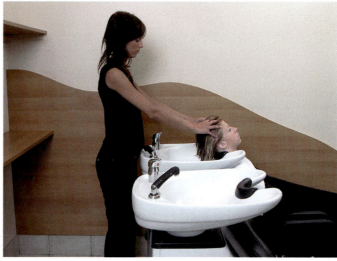

Figure 8.21 Posture

Describe what would be good posture at the washbasin:

Removal of colour

The three descriptions listed here detail the procedure for removing different types of colour from hair. Review the previous chapter and then give each description its correct title.

It is important to emulsify the hairline. This will make it easier to remove the colour from the skin. To do this, massage the area using your fingertips. An emulsion will then be formed which can be rinsed away. Rinse the hair starting with the forehead, then move on to the sides of the head and finally through the lengths. Dispense the shampoo into the palm of the hand, gently rub both hands together to evenly distribute the shampoo through the hair. Apply to the hair. Use the amount of shampoo as recommended by the manufacturer. Do not use more than the recommended amount. Massage the shampoo into the head and once the whole area is covered, rinse. The water temperature and pressure must be tested with the client. If the stylist has asked for two washes, then repeat this procedure. Condition the hair with a suitable conditioner as instructed by the stylist. Rinse off. Remove excess moisture with a gentle towel-through.

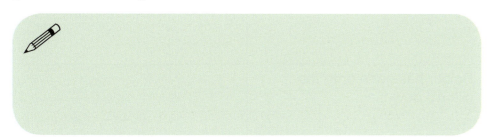

This type of colour must just be rinsed away. There is no need to condition as the colouring products have conditioning properties contained within them.

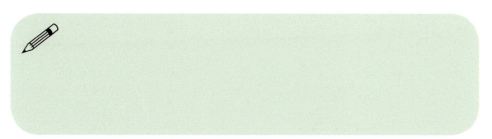

Carefully unfold each of these before removal. Product should be rinsed from each individual one.

Problems during colour rinsing

This table shows you the problems that occur during the rinsing process. Fill in the right hand column. Start by noting down the action that you THINK you should take and then review the previous chapter. Add any additional notes that you think will be useful.

Problem	Action
Colour from foils or highlights is leaking onto to other parts of the hair	
Colour has gone into the client's eye	
Colour still on hair after rinsing	
Client's skin has colour on	
Colour has gone onto the client's gown	

8.4 Assessment

Well done! If you have studied all the content of this unit you may be ready to test your knowledge.

Check out the 'Preparing for assessments' section in Chapter 1 if you have not already done so and always remember:

- You can only do your best if you have . . .
  - studied hard
  - completed the activities
  - completed the worksheets
  - practised, practised, practised
  - and then revised!

Now carry out the online multiple-choice quiz

. . . and good luck in the final exam, which will be arranged by your tutor/assessor.

Top tips

The most important attribute to have when working as a hairdresser is excellent communication and customer service skills. You may be an amazing hairdresser, but if you do not make your clients feel valued and comfortable, they will not come back to you.
Lindsay Bellis, Lecturer in Hairdressing and Bridal Hair at Yale College

Health and safety

Following health and safety legislation shows your clients and employer that you take your job seriously.
Samantha Raybould, Yale College, Wrexham

Create a positive impression

Think like a client; would you rather walk through the door of a salon where everyone looks miserable or happy?
Carly Embling-Loxton, Helen Ward and Linda Powell, Swindon College

When you greet a client for the first time, don't be afraid to shake their hand when you introduce yourself. It's professional and shows confidence, which all clients look for in a hair stylist.
Samantha Raybould, Yale College, Wrexham

Advise and consult

Sit next to the client, at eye level, when carrying out a consultation. This will stop the client feeling intimidated by you standing over them and will also help you talk to them face to face rather than through the mirror, as although this is normal to hairdressers, clients may feel uncomfortable.
Mandy Durkin, Saks Education

As well as asking your client what they *would* like, also ask them what they *do not* like.
Carly Embling-Loxton, Helen Ward and Linda Powell, Swindon College

Reception duties

Reception is your salon's 'first impression'. It must be clean, warm and welcoming and so must the people that are behind it!
Carly Embling-Loxton, Helen Ward and Linda Powell, Swindon College

Promote additional services or products

Never assume that your client wants 'the usual'. Always tell them about new products, services and techniques available in your

salon. Even if they are not wanted they will be happy that you have offered.
Carly Embling-Loxton, Helen Ward and Linda Powell, Swindon College

Effectiveness at work

Being able to recognise your salon's unique selling point is vital for success within the hair and beauty industry.
Karen Wright, Head of School Hair and Beauty Therapy, Runshaw College

When creating your own 'look book', give your signature services names to highlight your individuality as a hairdresser. For example, 'hidden lights' is a lowlighting technique used to complement the client's natural depth and tone.
Andrea Larter, Hairdressing Lecturer at Redbridge College

Shampoo, condition and treat the hair and scalp

A scalp massage whilst conditioning is normally the part of the service that the client enjoys the most, so make sure your technique keeps them coming back for more!
Carly Embling-Loxton, Helen Ward and Linda Powell, Swindon College

Style and finish hair

When styling long hair that is thick and heavy, secure it up to the crown area using small bands, then design your curls around this. Hair will stay in place for longer and it will stop the hair sagging.
Sue Sweeny, A. P. & Section Leader for hairdressing, Chichester College

Only apply serum to the mid lengths and ends of thick/dense hair. Doing this will avoid oily roots.
Sarah Flecknor, Hairdressing Tutor, Graduate Salon, Grimsby Institute and University Centre

Give every client a 'commentary' of the way you are blow-drying their hair and the products/tools you are using. This way they are much more likely to be able to recreate the look at home.
Mandy Durkin, Saks Education

Always show your client the back of their hair before you apply hairspray. If they aren't happy with the finish it will be harder to change once the hairspray is on.
Carly Embling-Loxton, Helen Ward and Linda Powell, Swindon College

Use a few Velcro rollers around the crown when the hair is still warm from blow-drying. This will give added lift, and can then be secured in place with a little hairspray.
Vanda Dean, Graduate Salon, Grimsby Institute and University Centre

Straightening irons are not only for styling hair poker straight. Think of them as styling irons, experiment with different styles creating waves, curls and root lift on styles. You can even use them for pin curling.
Lindsay Bellis, Lecturer in Hairdressing and Bridal Hair at Yale College

Set and dress hair

With any setting technique, always allow the hair to cool prior to removing the rollers. This will ensure a nice firm result with a shiny finish and it will help to avoid static.
David Rabjohns, East Surrey College

Be sure not to leave any gaps amongst your rollers as it will leave gaps in the hair once dry.
Carly Embling-Loxton, Helen Ward and Linda Powell, Swindon College

Never open grips and pins in your mouth; this is unhygienic and could cause cross infection.
Natalie Stephens, Hairdressing Level 2 and Level 3 Curriculum Leader, Creative Academies, Gloucestershire College

When you have spent hours putting someone's hair up for an occasion, advise them that if they are having a bath in the evening, to run the cold water first before adding warm water, as this neutralises steam and stops their hair dropping (the hydrogen bonds will not break).
Carly Embling-Loxton, Helen Ward and Linda Powell, Swindon College

When dry setting the hair with Velcro rollers, spritz the ends with a light volume spray. This will make the ends easier to wrap around the roller, smooth the ends and will make the set last longer.
Lindsay Bellis, Lecturer in Hairdressing and Bridal Hair at Yale College

Cutting hair

Right-handed people tend to cut base lines that slope longer towards the left. This is due to the fact that the direction we cut in is from right to left (and vice versa for left-handed people). Knowing this makes it easier to self-correct the cutting angle and create even and balanced base lines.
David Rabjohns, East Surrey College

When performing a one length cut *always* ensure the client's head is looking down towards the floor. This will prevent graduation on the perimeter line.
Paula Shaw, Lecturer – Hairdressing, Knowsley Community College

When cutting hair, always make sure your client's legs are uncrossed to prevent the cut becoming unbalanced.
Abby Crowhurst, Divisional Lead Manager Hair & Beauty, The Manchester College

Remember the fringe is the part of the haircut the client will see the most, so pay particular attention to this area when cutting. It will define your cut.
Mandy Durkin, Saks Education

When cutting a one length style, try to keep the cutting line at eye level. On very long hair this may require asking your client to stand.
Virginia Collins, Graduate Salon, Grimsby Institute and University Centre

When cutting, don't be scared to turn your client around in their chair so they are sideways to the mirror; that way you can check whether you are elevating your sections enough or not.
Nicki Chaplin, Graduate Salon, Grimsby Institute and University Centre

When carrying out a cut, ensure that you always have a water bottle to hand before you start. The hair should be wet at all times; this creates even tension and makes the hair easier to work with.
Lindsay Bellis, Lecturer in Hairdressing and Bridal Hair at Yale College

When cutting hair, make the most use of your tools and equipment. Use your mirror to continuously check your client's and your own posture and how you are angling, sectioning and cutting the hair. You should also think of your comb as a ruler, using it to help you achieve your required angles.
Lindsay Bellis, Lecturer in Hairdressing and Bridal Hair at Yale College

Colour hair

Never wash your tint bowl up until the service is over. Tint removes tint from the client's skin and can also be used if any touch-ups are needed rather than mix up more products!
Zoe Grimes, Assessor, Redbridge College

When you have finished weaving a full head of bleach foils application, take small strips of cotton wool and put one between each foil at the root area. This will prevent any seepage from touching the scalp when the bleach expands during development.
Susie Phillips, Lead Personal Learning Advisor, Redbridge College

When choosing a colour for a client always check their eye colour and skin tone as these will tell you whether your client would suit a cool or warm tone colour.
Sue Sweeny, A. P. & Section Leader for hairdressing, Chichester College

When describing colours to clients always use terms that a client can relate to such as 'honey highlights' or 'chocolate'.
Suzanne Szepeta, Vision West Notts

As well as using antioxy between colour processes, condition the hair. This will keep it in optimum condition and will give an improved colour result.
Janice Yardley, Graduate Salon, Grimsby Institute and University Centre

When diluting peroxide, always do so at eye level and on a flat surface, using eye protection.
Nicki Chaplin, Graduate Salon, Grimsby Institute and University Centre

Perm and neutralise hair

After applying your perm lotion, change your cotton wool after five minutes. If you do not change the cotton wool, most of the excess will have dripped through and will be lying against the client's skin.
Carly Embling-Loxton, Helen Ward and Linda Powell, Swindon College

Plait and twist hair

If hair is too clean and slippery to work with, lightly spray some hairspray through it to give it some grip.
Carly Embling-Loxton, Helen Ward and Linda Powell, Swindon College

Cut facial hair to shape

Moustaches can be worn as part of the beard, or as a separate entity. Likewise, sideburns can also be integrated or separate from a beard.
Dawn Buttle, Academy Manager, Salon Services, Hairdressing, South Essex College of Further and Higher Education

Glossary

This glossary is also available online at www.atthairdressing.com where you can search for important words and phrases and even translate them into other languages.

We have added a guide to the pronunciation (proh-nun-see-ay-shun) of unusual words in this format at the front of the book.

Abrasion	*An area of the skin which has worn away.*
Absorbed	*Taken in through the surface of an object.*
Accessories	*Jewellery or other items worn in the hair.*
Accident	*A mishap that can often lead to injury.*
Account	*A record of financial transactions.*
Accuracy	*How close the data given is to the true value.*
Accurate	*Exact.*
Acetic acid	*Used in acid rinses (vinegar rinse).*
Acid balanced	*Lotion with the same pH as the skin (4.5–5.5).*
Acid	*A solution with a pH of less than 7.*
Action plan	*A method of outlining steps and actions in order achieve a particular goal.*
Adapt	*To suit another purpose.*
Added hair	*Extensions and hairpieces.*
Additional media	*Materials other than ornamentation used for creating a look (i.e. accessories, make-up and clothes).*
Additive	*Substance added to improve a product.*
Adequate	*Sufficient.*
Adhere	*To stick to.*
Adhesions	*Scar tissue.*
Advertising	*Promoting products or services.*
Advice	*Guidance offered by someone.*
Afro comb	*Comb to detangle afro or curly hair.*
Afro	*Type of hair.*
Aftercare	*Continuing service given to the client.*
Agitation	*To keep a substance or object moving.*
Alcohol	*Solvent used in setting lotions.*
Alcoholics Anonymous	*A worldwide group of men and women who meet in order to help one another stop drinking alcohol and remain sober.*
Alkaline	*Solution with a pH above 7.*
Allergic reaction	*Abnormal reaction to a substance.*
Allergy	*Abnormal reaction to a substance.*
Almond oil	*Vegetable oil used for hot oil scalp treatments. Ingredient of control creams.*
Alopecia areata	*Balding condition made up of small round patches which often follow the line of a nerve.*
Alopecia	*A general term meaning baldness.*

Alpha keratin	*Hair in its natural unstretched state.*
Alphabetical	*In the order of the letters of the alphabet.*
Alter	*To change.*
Alternative	*A choice.*
Amino-acid	*The component units of protein.*
Ammonia	*Colourless fluid used as a solvent.*
Anagen	*During the period of active growth the hair is said to be in anagen.*
Analyse	*Examine in detail (i.e. the condition of the hair).*
Androgenic alopecia	*Hereditary male pattern baldness.*
Annual Income	*Amount of money you earn each year.*
Annual	*Yearly.*
Anonymous	*To be unknown.*
Antiseptic	*A substance which prevents the multiplication of germs but does not necessarily kill them. Examples are cetrimide and chloroxylenol.*
Antivirus software	*A software package that prevents computer viruses from damaging or destroying the system.*
Appeal	*To ask urgently.*
Appearance	*The way that somebody looks.*
Application	*Another name for a computer program such as Microsoft Word.*
Appointment	*A specified time for a meeting.*
Appraisal	*A system of reviewing an employee's job performance carried out by the employee and employer.*
Area	*Length x width.*
Artificial	*To be man-made.*
Assemble	*To gather together.*
Assess	*To judge the condition (of hair).*
Assessor	*The candidate's teacher or tutor, who assesses the portfolio of evidence.*
Assistance	*Help.*
Asymmetric	*Unbalanced profile.*
Attract	*To draw an object or substance closer.*
Authorisation	*Agreed by the supervisor.*
Autoclave	*Apparatus used for sterilising tools, it works on the same principle as the pressure cooker.*
Avant-garde	*A term used to describe artwork that breaks away from tradition.*
Average	*The sum divided by the number of items.*
Awarding body	*There are several awarding bodies, for example City and Guilds, AQA, Edexcel and OCR.*
Back brushing	*Achieves a soft effect and will 'fluff' the hair with more bounce.*
Back combing	*Achieves a stiff style.*
Backup	*A second copy of work in case the original is damaged or destroyed. Should be stored away from the computer.*
Backwash	*Flow of water directed backwards.*
Bacteria	*Disease causing micro-organisms.*
Balance	*Equal distribution.*
Bands of colour	*Areas of the hair that appear lighter or darker than the rest of the hair.*
Barbicide	*Chemical used to sterilise tools.*

Barrel curl	*Used on very short hair to achieve the same result as rollers.*
Barrier cream	*A cream used to protect skin from contact with products.*
Barrier	*Something that blocks things from going past it.*
Base colour	*The client's natural hair colour.*
Baseline	*Lowest point and foundation of haircut.*
Basic skills	*Reading, writing, speaking in English (or Welsh) and using numbers sufficiently well to be able to function in society and at work. Key skills and basic skills overlap at levels 1 and 2.*
Basin	*A sink. Used to wash clients hair.*
Beta keratin	*The stretched (wet) state of hair.*
Biased	*Favouring one thing over another.*
Bicarbonate	*Mineral of hard water.*
Binds	*Ties to.*
Bleach	*Chemical used to lighten (whiten) hair colour by oxidisation.*
Blending	*Combining two sections.*
Block colouring technique	*Colouring the hair in a large area.*
Blow drying	*The method of drying the hair using a hand dryer.*
Bluetooth	*Wireless Technology. A chip is responsible for the transmission of data between a wide range of devices (mobile phone and hands-free system) through short range digital two-way radio.*
Bob	*A one length hair cut.*
Body language	*Refers to facial expressions, gestures or a particular way a person is standing. Non-verbal communication.*
Brick cutting	*A technique of texturising by cutting small parts of hair in a 'brick' fashion.*
Brickwork	*Term used for positioning rollers correctly.*
Brittle	*Hair that can be easily broken.*
Buckled	*To be out of shape.*
Budget	*A list of incomings and outgoings used in financial planning.*
Burdock root oil	*Used in shampoos for dry scalp.*
Calcium	*Mineral affecting the hardness of water.*
Canities	*Pigmentation cells not functioning, hair turns white.*
Capability	*The ability to complete a task.*
Cape	*Waterproof gown used to protect client's clothes.*
Capillary	*Very thin blood vessel.*
Career Prospect	*The direction in which your career could move.*
Cash	*Money, banknotes and coins.*
Catagen	*Stage of hair growth: hair falls out, follicle shrinks.*
CD-ROM	*Compact Disc Read Only Memory. Stores up to 800Mb of data. The data is 'read only' which means that you cannot change or overwrite it.*
Ceramic	*An object that is made into a shape, then hardened using heat.*
Cetrimide	*Antiseptic chemical used for* pityriasis capitis.
Characteristic	*A feature or quality of a person, place or thing.*
Checking	*Hair has a balanced front, sides, sections match.*
Cheque guarantee card	*Guarantee by bank for payment of the order.*
Cheque	*Written order to bank for payment.*
Chip and PIN	*Customers key in a PIN at point of sale instead of signing a receipt.*

Chlorinated water	*Water with added chlorine, can damage the hair.*
Cicatrical alopecia	*Baldness caused by physical/chemical damage to skin.*
Circular brush	*Used to loosen out the set or achieve a softer look.*
Circumference	*The boundary line of a circle.*
Clarify	*To make clear.*
Clarifying	*To make clear.*
Classic	*A look that will not age.*
Client suggestion box	*A box used by clients to post written feedback.*
Climazone	*Equipment to dry hair and speed chemical processes.*
Clipboard	*A temporary area used to store copied information.*
Clipper over comb	*Technique for cutting hair. Clippers are used to cut hair following the movement over a comb.*
Clock spring curls	*Tight curls or wave movements.*
Clockwise	*To move in the same direction as the hands on a clock.*
Closed question	*A question with a definite answer (i.e. yes/no).*
Club cutting	*Hair cut straight across.*
Coal tar	*Chemical with antiseptic qualities.*
Coarse hair	*Hair with a thick shaft.*
Coconut	*Used in shampoos for dry scalps.*
Colleagues	*The people that you work with.*
Collodion	*A syrupy, clean solution of pyroxylin, alcohol and ether.*
Colour correction	*The way in which hair colour or bleach problems are corrected.*
Colour reducer	*A product used to remove permanent hair colour.*
Colour reduction	*A product used to remove permanent colour from the hair.*
Colour star	*Colour chart to achieve desired colour.*
Colour test	*Test used to monitor colour development.*
Colour tone	*Warm/cool shades of colour tints.*
Commitment	*To bind yourself to a certain action.*
Communicate	*To exchange information.*
Communication	*An exchange of thoughts and information.*
Complementary skills	*Skills other than hairdressing but nonetheless essential.*
Comprehensive	*To cover a wide area.*
Compression ratio	*The volume above the piston when it is at BDC compared to the volume above the piston when it is at TDC.*
Compulsory	*Must be completed.*
Computer application	*Programs such as Word, Excel and PowerPoint.*
Computer crash	*An event that causes the computer to become inactive. This can often result in the loss of unsaved work.*
Computerised	*Performed by using a computer.*
Concave	*To curve inwards.*
Concentrated	*A liquid that has had its dilution reduced.*
Concise	*Expressing a lot but in few words.*
Condition	*Reference to the state of the hair's health.*
Conditioner	*Product used to enhance hair condition.*
Confidence	*A feeling of trust.*
Confidential Information	*Information that is private and should be protected.*

Confidentiality	*To keep secret.*
Confirm	*To make more firm by repeating.*
Constricted	*Made smaller than normal.*
Constructive	*To improve.*
Consultation	*Discuss individual needs with the client.*
Contagious	*Infection can be transferred by contact.*
Contamination	*Spread of disease by contact of non-sterile objects.*
Contradictory	*To oppose in disagreement.*
Contraindication	*A condition preventing a treatment.*
Contribution	*To give.*
Conventional	*Ordinary.*
Conversion factor	*Used to make it easier when converting from one form of 'measurement' to another.*
Conversions	*To change one expression to another. For example, expressing miles in kilometres.*
Convex	*To curve outwards.*
Cool shade	*Colours such as blue.*
Co-operative	*To join in and help others in your team.*
Cornrows	*Braids that are plaited close to the scalp.*
Cortex	*Middle layer of the hair shaft.*
Courteous	*To be polite.*
Cowlick	*Growth pattern of the hair.*
Creative	*To be artistic.*
Credit	*System of allowing customers to pay later for services.*
Creeping oxidation	*Active product left on the hair separating the cuticle plates.*
Crimping iron	*Tool used for crimping the hair.*
Crocodile clamps	*Used to hold hair while sectioning.*
Cross check	*Checking haircut.*
Cross-infection	*The spreading of infection between individuals and objects.*
Cross-section	*The area exposed if a cut were to be made through the centre of an object.*
Crown	*The top of the head.*
Crucial	*Very important.*
Curl rearranger	*The product used in the first step of a two-step perm.*
Curling tongs	*Used for curling the hair.*
Curling	*To form curls in the hair.*
Currency	*A unit of exchange used as a form of money.*
Current	*A look that is fashionable.*
Cut throat razor	*Used for tapering wet hair and shaving.*
Cuticle	*Outer layer of the hair shaft.*
Cysteine	*An amino acid joined by sulphur bonds.*
Cystine	*An amino acid joined by sulphur bonds.*
Damaged cuticle	*Cuticle scale open, absorbs moisture.*
Data Protection Act	*An Act that provides rights for individuals regarding the obtaining, use, holding and disclosure of information about themselves.*
Debit card	*A card guarantee that a debit will be honoured by the bank.*
Debit	*Cash deducted from a customer's account.*

Decimal place	*The position of numbers after (to the right of) the decimal point.*
Decimal	*A number system that uses a base of 10.*
Decomposition	*The breakdown of a material.*
Defamatory	*Untrue and harmful information.*
Denman brush	*A type of brush used for achieving a thorough brush.*
Dense	*Thick.*
Depth	*The natural lightness/darkness of the hair.*
Dermal papilla	*Situated at the hair follicle base, supplying all the materials needed for growth.*
Dermatitis	*Abnormal skin condition.*
Dermis	*Lower layer of the skin.*
Design plan	*A document used for planning a project outlining objectives, budget, roles and responsibilities, resources, health and safety issue etc.*
Design	*The arrangement of elements.*
Designated	*To have been selected for a task or duty.*
Detergent	*Cleaning substance used in shampoos.*
Determine	*To decide.*
Dexterity	*To perform tasks with the hands, using skill.*
Diagnose	*Identify the problem, need or want.*
Diameter	*The line that goes through the centre of the circle.*
Dictionary	*A book containing a list of words in alphabetical order. Each word has information given about it (i.e., the definition).*
Diet	*Nutrient content and food calorific value.*
Diffuse alopecia	*Condition in which the hair thins gradually.*
Diffuser	*Attachment to a dryer for special effect.*
Digit	*A number.*
Dilute	*Weaken the concentration (strength) of a solution.*
Disconnected	*A type of haircut featuring different lengths without being blended together.*
Discriminatory	*Unfair or unequal treatment of a person due to their age, sex, disability, race, religion etc.*
Disk drives	*The primary data storage device used by computers. It stores and retrieves data.*
Dispense	*To give out.*
Disposable	*Designed to be thrown away after use.*
Dissatisfied	*Not happy.*
Distribute	*Spread out.*
Distributed	*Spread out.*
Di-sulphide bond	*Sulphur link of two cystine amino-acids.*
Dizziness	*A spinning sensation.*
Double base-line	*Working (cutting) on an extra line over a shorter one.*
Double booking	*Two treatments scheduled at the same time.*
Double crown	*A growth pattern where the crowns jump and swirl in opposite directions.*
Dressing hair	*The way in which hair is finished using different techniques (i.e. smoothing or curling).*
Dressing out brush	*Brush that has a rubber base for more gentle brushing.*
Dressing out	*Styling hair.*
Droop	*To sag, or hang loosely.*
Dry setting	*Hair is altered temporarily using heated rollers.*

Dryer	*Equipment for drying hair, can be hand-held or floor standing.*
Duty	*Something that you are obliged to do.*
Effect	*The consequence of.*
Effective	*To work well.*
Efficient	*To get the job done with little waste of time or energy.*
Effleurage	*Smooth stroking massage movement, using palm of the hand.*
EFTPOS	*Electronic Point of Sale.*
Elasticity test	*Test used to assess damage to cortex of hair.*
Eliminate	*To remove.*
E-mail	*Electronic Mail. Messages sent from one person to another electronically via a computer.*
Emergency services	*Fire, Ambulance, Police.*
Emerging	*A look that is nearly in fashion.*
Emoticons	*A way of expressing emotions in online communication. E.g., :-).*
Emotion	*State of feeling, associated with stress, which can affect the condition of the hair.*
Empathise	*To understand someone else's feelings.*
Emulsify	*To blend two liquids that wouldn't naturally combine together.*
Emulsifying agent	*To blend two liquids that wouldn't naturally combine together.*
Emulsion bleach	*Type of bleach used for full head treatment.*
Emulsion	*A mixture of two or more liquids that do not blend together.*
Enhance	*To make the best of.*
Enquiry	*A question.*
Ensure	*To make certain.*
Epidermis	*Outer layer of the skin.*
Equal opportunities	*Everyone to be given equal rights.*
Equipment	*An instrument.*
Establish	*To find out.*
Estimate	*To guess, but based on experience!*
Ethical	*Morally correct.*
Eumelanin	*Black and brown pigments.*
Evacuate	*To remove.*
Evaluate	*To assess.*
Evidence	*This is what a candidate needs to produce to prove they have the skills required.*
Exaggerate	*To emphasise.*
Exerting	*To use or apply.*
Exhibition	*An event that products and services are advertised and sold.*
Expire	*To finish.*
Expression	*A way to communicate.*
Extension	*An additional set of numbers that connects to the same telephone line.*
External assessment	*A test set externally to check portfolio evidence.*
Extinguish	*To put out.*
Fatigue	*Tiredness: can be caused by poor working posture.*
Faulty	*Does not work.*
Feasible	*To be capable of being achieved.*
Feathering	*Technique used to remove volume or length of hair.*

Feature	*A characteristic of a person's face.*
Feedback	*The opinions of others or yourself concerned with a product or service.*
Filing system	*Method of keeping records of client treatments.*
Financial	*Monetary.*
Fine hair	*Term used to describe thin or delicate hair strands.*
Fine pins	*Equipment used to secure pin curls or dress hair up.*
Finger drying	*To dry hair using a hairdryer and your hands.*
Finger waving	*Technique where hair is moulded into an 's' shape using fingers and comb. Also known as water waving.*
Finishing spray	*A product that holds hair in place and protects against weather and humidity.*
Fire extinguisher	*A device for putting out small fires.*
Fixing	*Alternative name for neutralising hair.*
Flamboyant	*To be excessively ornamented.*
Flammable	*Can catch fire.*
Flat brush	*A brush used for smoothing the hair. Also known as spiral brush.*
Flexible	*Being able to accept change.*
Floppy Disk	*A portable disk that stores 1.44 Mb of information.*
Focused	*To the point.*
Foils	*Thin sheets of metal generally used for highlighting/lowlighting hair.*
Follicle	*Sac containing the hair shaft in the epidermis.*
Folliculitis	*Bacterial infection of the follicle.*
Forgery	*A copy that is illegal.*
Fractions	*A number of parts out of another number of parts.*
Fragilitas crinium	*Hair splits at the ends and along the shaft.*
Fraud	*The act of deceiving to obtain money.*
Freehand cutting	*Cutting without tension.*
Friction massage	*Used during shampooing to work from the front of the scalp to the nape using the pads of the fingers in a vigorous movement.*
Fungi	*Parasitic organisms that do not contain chlorophyll. Includes mushrooms and yeast.*
Gel	*Lotion used to make hair spiky or stand-up.*
General Practitioner	*A doctor.*
Gesture	*A hand or body motion.*
Glare	*Reflection from the sun or a light onto the computer screen making it difficult to see properly.*
Gloss	*Lotion used to make hair look shiny.*
Goals	*Objectives relating to a particular time. Can be short-term or long-term.*
Google	*Popular search engine.*
Gown	*Protective garment used to cover clients' clothes.*
Gradient	*The degree of incline.*
Graduation	*The shape of a style created by cutting hair to achieve a look where the inner length is longer than the outer length.*
Grammar	*Forming well written, easy to read sentences, paragraphs and documents with the use of punctuation (i.e., full stops, commas etc.).*
Grievance	*To have felt grief after a wrong doing has occurred. A formal complaint.*
Growth pattern	*The direction of the hair growth.*

Guideline	*Mesh of hair used to measure other sections.*
Hair balance	*Profile shape of the hair style.*
Hair extensions	*Additional pieces of hair attached to current hair.*
Hair shaft	*The part of the hair that is above the skin.*
Hair straighteners	*Heated styling equipment designed to straighten the hair. Can also be used for other styling techniques.*
Hair structure	*The microscopic make up of hair.*
Hairline	*Natural hairline around the neck and face.*
Hairspray	*A product that holds hair in place and protects against weather and humidity.*
Hard disk	*A storage device that holds large amounts of data.*
Hard water	*Water with increased levels of calcium, requires more soap and detergent, forms scum.*
Hardware	*The physical components of a computer system.*
Hazard	*A source of danger.*
Hazardous	*Involving risk or danger.*
Heart shape	*Face shape for which suitable hairstyles include a fringe and hair between ear and jaw.*
Heat protectors	*Products applied to prevent the hair becoming damaged from heated styling equipment.*
Heated rollers	*Creates volume root lift, curl and hair direction.*
Heated tongs	*An electrical device used to curl hair.*
Henna	*Permanent vegetable tint.*
Hereditary	*Passed on from parents (genetic).*
Herpes simplex	*A viral infection affecting the skin and nervous system.*
Hexachlorophene	*Chemical used with antiseptic properties used on dry scalp.*
Hierarchy	*A group of people ranked in order of job position.*
Highlights	*Lightening strands of hair.*
Hinder	*To prevent something.*
Hologram	*A 3-D image.*
Hood dryer	*Floor-mounted dryer, creates an overall even drying effect quickly.*
Hormone	*Chemical produced by the body controlling chemical reactions in the body.*
Hospitality	*The way in which a client is welcomed and received into the salon.*
Hostility	*Unfriendly.*
Humidity	*The dampness in the hair.*
Hydrogen bond	*A chemical bonding linking oxygen to hydrogen to form water.*
Hydrogen peroxide	*An agent used for oxidising when colouring and perming.*
Hydrogen	*Flammable gas occurring in water and ammonia.*
Hydrophilic	*Will mix with water.*
Hydrophobic	*Will not mix with water (repelled).*
Hygiene	*Principles and practice of sanitation to ensure good health.*
Hygroscopic	*Absorbs moisture.*
ICT	*Information and Communication Technology.*
Identify	*To consider.*
Image	*A perception of (hair salon's image).*
Immiscible	*Liquids that are incapable of being mixed together.*
Imperial measurement	*Defined by three measures – the gallon, the yard and the pound.*

Impetigo	*Contagious bacterial skin disease.*
Impression	*Outward appearance.*
Incapacitated	*A person with a mental, emotional or physical impairment.*
Incoming telephone call	*To receive a telephone call.*
Incompatibility test	*Method of detecting products used in previous treatments that may contra-react.*
Incompatible	*Cannot be used with (other chemicals).*
Incorporating	*To include.*
Infection	*A disease caused by micro-organisms.*
Infectious	*The spreading of disease.*
Infestation	*A group of parasites.*
Infirm	*A person lacking in strength.*
Inflation	*The general increase in the price of goods and services.*
Ingest	*Take in the body by the mouth.*
Ingredient	*Part of.*
Inhalation	*Take into the body through the airways.*
Initial and diagnostic assessment	*This is carried out to find a candidate's strengths and weaknesses, current levels of attainment and potential.*
Initiative	*To take the first step.*
Innovative	*To be forward thinking in terms of ideas and themes.*
Input device	*A device that allows you to put information into the computer (e.g. keyboard, mouse).*
Interactive	*Two-way communication.*
Internal shape	*Internal shape of the haircut.*
Internal verification	*The process whereby a centre ensures it operates consistently and to national standards in interpreting and assessing the key skills.*
Internal	*Inside.*
Internet	*A worldwide network of computers that allows us to view the World Wide Web.*
Interpersonal skills	*The ability to deal well with several different people.*
Interpret	*To understand and be able to explain something.*
Interpreted	*To make sense of.*
Inter-quartile mean	*The average of the values in the inter-quartile range.*
Inter-quartile range	*The range of numbers with the upper and lower quartiles removed.*
Inter-twining	*To twist together.*
Intimidating	*To make somebody feel uncomfortable, timid or even fearful.*
Inversion	*Create a concave shape in the hair.*
Inward nape	*Nape hair grows strongly to the centre.*
Irritant	*A chemical that can cause irritation or inflammation to the skin.*
Irritate	*To annoy or cause discomfort.*
IT	*Information Technology.*
Itemise	*To list individually.*
Job description	*A set of responsibilities given by an employer for a particular job.*
Journal	*Day-by-day diary or similar.*
Keloid	*Irregular fibrous tissue, which is formed at the place of a scar or injury.*
Keratin	*Protein that makes up hair. Contains large amounts of sulphur.*
Key data	*Important, relevant information.*

Keyboard	*The typewriter-like keys used to input data into a computer. An input device.*
Knowledge	*To know something.*
Lanolin	*Product used in shampoos used for a dry scalp.*
Lanugo	*Foetal body hair.*
Latent heat	*Body heat from the scalp.*
Layering	*Hair cut at various angles.*
Legislation	*A law.*
Libellous	*Untrue and harmful information.*
Library	*Collection of materials (i.e. books or CDs).*
Lice	*Nits, insects that infest the hair.*
Lift pic	*Root lift achieved by setting rollers on the section.*
Lift	*Lightening the hair colour.*
Lightening	*To remove colour from the hair.*
Lime scale	*Deposit of bicarbonates caused by boiling water.*
Long shape	*Face shape suited by fuller sides hairstyle and flatter on top.*
Lotion	*Product that has the consistency of a light cream.*
Lower quartile	*Data is split into four equal quarters. The lowest quarter is referred to as the lower quartile. For example the lower quartile of 100 is the lowest 25 of the numbers.*
Lowlights	*Sections of hair that have been toned darker than the full head of hair.*
Magnesium	*Mineral affecting the hardness of the water.*
Maintain	*To keep something at a specific level.*
Maintenance	*To care for.*
Manoeuvre	*To move.*
Manual	*Not computerised.*
Mapping	*Used to identify opportunities for developing and assessing key skills within the curriculum.*
Marcel iron	*Equipment used for setting hair.*
Marketing	*The method of advertising, promoting and selling to customers.*
Massage	*Manipulative movement using the fingers and palms of the hand.*
Master card	*Type of credit card.*
MB	*Megabyte. Used to measure computer memory. 1 Mb = 1,000,000 bytes or 1024 Kb (kilobytes).*
Mean	*The average value (the sum divided by the number of items).*
Median	*The middle number of a series when the data is arranged in ascending order.*
Medicated	*Contains healing or medical additives.*
Medium hair	*Hair shaft is middle-range in size.*
Medulla	*The central part of the hair shaft.*
Melanin	*Colouring pigment of the hair.*
Melanocytes	*A cell that contains the pigment melanin.*
Memory chip	*A chip that stores data.*
Merchandise	*Goods that are to be sold.*
Merely	*No more than.*
Meshes	*Smaller sections of main sections.*
Method	*The way in which a task is carried out.*
Methodically	*To work through something in the correct order.*

Metric measurement	*A system designed to regulate measurement. Each quantity has a single unit. These include; metre, kilogramme, ampere.*
Micro-organisms	*Tiny forms of life, only seen through a microscope.*
Microphone	*A device that converts sound waves to audio signals.*
Microsoft Office	*A package of programs including Word Processor (Word), Spreadsheet (Excel), Presentation (PowerPoint), Email and Organisation (Outlook).*
Misconception	*To have a thought that is incorrect.*
Mobility	*Movement.*
Mode	*The most common number in a series.*
Modifications	*Changes made.*
Moisturise	*Add or restore moisture to the hair.*
Molecule	*Chemical unit of two or more atoms.*
Monilethrix	*Uneven production of cells in dermal papilla causing brittle hair.*
Monitor	*The screen that displays information produced on a computer. An output device.*
Moulding	*To sculpture the hair.*
Mouse	*An input device that allows the user to move the pointer around the screen and click on different items to operate computer applications.*
Mousse foam	*Lotion used for setting hair.*
Multiple choice	*A selection of answers.*
Nape	*Lowest point of hair growth at the back of the head.*
Natural base	*Natural colour of the hair.*
Natural parting	*A natural parting where the hair falls making a dividing line.*
Navigation	*The way in which you get around a program or website.*
Negative communication	*A comment or statement expressing lack of approval.*
Negative ions	*Electrically charged atoms.*
Network card	*A piece of hardware that allows computers to be connected to a network.*
Network	*Interlinked group of computers so that resources can be shared.*
Neutralise	*Fixing the structure of the hair after permanent waving or relaxing.*
Nitro-dyes	*Semi-permanent colouring dyes.*
Non-contagious	*Infection that cannot be transferred by contact.*
Non-verbal	*Any form of communication that does not use words (i.e. traffic lights, shaking somebody's hand and smiling).*
Normalising	*Alternative word for neutralising.*
Nozzle	*Attachment for dryer to achieve a special effect.*
Objective information	*Information that is unbiased and open minded.*
Objectives	*The goals to be achieved.*
Obligatory	*Compulsory.*
Obscene	*Offensive, foul, disgusting.*
Obstacles	*Objects that are in the way.*
Occipital bone	*Convex protruding bone at the back of the skull.*
Occupation	*The job that you do. For example, training to be a motor mechanic is training for an occupation.*
Odour	*Smell or fragrance.*
Offensive	*To attack somebody/something by words or physically.*
Office Applications	*A package of programs including Word Processor (Word), Spreadsheet (Excel), Presentation (PowerPoint), Email and Organisation (Outlook).*

One length cut	*Hair cut in a 'bob'.*
Open centred pin curls	*Loose, soft pin curls.*
Open question	*A question used to allow the respondent to expand on their answer.*
Opinion	*A personal belief.*
Organisms	*A life form made of a complex system of cells and tissues.*
Ornamentation	*Decoration to be added to hair once it has been styled.*
Outgoing telephone call	*To make a telephone call to somebody.*
Output device	*A device that allows information from the computer to be displayed (e.g. monitor, printer).*
Outside shape	*Shape of the hair cut on the base line.*
Oval shape	*A perfect-shaped face to suit any hair style.*
Overlap	*Time of a treatment going into the time scheduled for another.*
Oxidation	*The addition of oxygen in a chemical reaction.*
Oxymelanin	*Melanin reduced by bleach.*
Packet	*An item used to colour hair in sections.*
Paddle brush	*Used for smoothing hair.*
Parasite	*An organism that feeds from and lives on another organism.*
Participate	*To take part in.*
Particle	*A tiny part of an object.*
Pear shape	*Face shape for which suitable hairstyles should have lots of volume around the temples but flat around the jaw line.*
Pediculosis capitis	*To be infected with lice on the scalp.*
Penetrate	*To enter.*
Penetrating conditioner	*Work by penetrating the cortex and help to repair damage by adding protein. They are known as substantive products.*
Percent	*The proportion of one part of something to the whole. Per means 'out of' and 'cent' means 'hundred'.*
Percentage change	*Changed amounts divided by the original value, then multiplied by 100.*
Performance criteria	*The standards from which you (the student) will be evaluated.*
Perimeter	*The sum of all the outside edges of a shape.*
Perm rod	*Rod around which hair is re-shaped.*
Permanent colour	*Colour containing molecules that penetrate the cuticle and are absorbed into the cortex. The tint remains until it is cut out.*
Perming	*The method of curling hair by altering the structure using chemicals.*
Petrissage	*A deep-kneading massage movement.*
pH	*Level of acidity/alkalinity.*
Pharmacist	*Somebody who carries out the service of preparing and distributing medicine.*
Pheomelanin	*Natural pigment of hair causing a red/yellow hair colour.*
Phrase	*A group of words in sequence.*
Pi	*3.141592 (3.142).*
Pigment	*Colour matter of the hair.*
Pin curling	*Open centre pin curl used to achieve loose flat look.*
Pine	*Product used in shampoos for dry scalp.*
Pityriasis capitis	*Continuous flaking of the epidermis (dandruff).*
Plagiarise	*Taking another person's work as your own.*
Plaiting	*Used to achieve a secure finish after dressing hair out.*

Planning	*The act of forming and following a programme to achieve a specific goal.*
Pleating	*Folds of hair secured with pins and grips.*
Pli	*Hair set in rollers or pin curls.*
Point to root	*Winding the hair from the ends of the hair to the root.*
Pointing	*Technique used to break up the points of the hair.*
Policy	*A plan of action.*
Polite	*To show regard to others. To use good manners.*
Polythene	*Lightweight plastic.*
Ponytail	*A hairstyle where the hair is drawn to the back of the head and secured with a band.*
Population of UK	*Number of people that live in the UK (about 60 Million in 2010).*
Porosity	*Ability to absorb moisture.*
Portfolio	*This is usually a folder that contains the evidence chosen to illustrate competence to satisfy individual key skills requirements.*
Positive communication	*A comment or statement expressing approval.*
Positive ions	*Electrically charged atoms.*
Posture	*Working position of the body.*
Potential	*Possibility that something may happen.*
Powder bleach	*Type of bleach used for highlights. Not usually recommended for full head.*
PPE	*Personal Protective Equipment. Equipment that is worn to protect people at work from risks to their health and safety.*
Precaution	*A method of reducing risk.*
Precise	*To be exact and accurate.*
Pre-colouring	*Applying a treatment to the hair before colouring, to improve the condition.*
Pre-perm shampoo	*Soapless detergent shampoo with no additives.*
Pre-perm test	*Detection of extent of curl from previous perm.*
Pre-pigmentation	*The method of adding a warm shade to the hair to replace missing pigments before re-colouring bleached hair.*
Presentation	*The way in which something is displayed.*
Pre-softening	*The application of a treatment to lift the cuticle from the hair allowing the colour to penetrate the cortex.*
Prevalent	*To be widespread.*
Pre-wrap lotion	*Method used to even out the porosity of hair.*
Pricing scanner	*A device that converts a visual form into a price.*
Prickly	*Sensation of cut hair next to client's skin.*
Primary colours	*Yellow, blue and red.*
Printer	*An output device that allows data from the computer to be displayed on paper.*
Probationary	*A trial period.*
Procedure	*A course of action.*
Processing time	*The length of time it takes for colour to develop.*
Processor	*The central processing unit oversees all of the other components of the system. Can be thought of as the brain of the computer.*
Product	*Items sold as part of the hair care process.*
Professional	*Term given to use of effective and efficient working methods.*
Profile	*Shape of the hair style.*
Profitable	*To obtain positive income from a transaction.*

Progress	*Positive development.*
Promotional	*To advertise or publicise.*
Promptly	*Straight away.*
Proportion	*The size of different parts in relation to each other.*
Props	*Items used for events.*
Protective gloves	*Rubber gloves used to protect hands from chemicals.*
Protective treatment	*Products used to stop damage to hair that has previously been treated. Applied before treatment.*
Protein	*Hair structure, made from amino acids.*
Protrude	*To stick out.*
Provenance	*The origins of information.*
PSI	*Pounds per square inch.*
Psoriasis	*Red patches on scalp covered by silver white scales.*
Pubic	*Type of terminal hair.*
Publicity	*To get attention for a product/service by advertising etc.*
Punctuation	*The use of marks and signs to form words, sentences, paragraphs etc.*
Qualified	*To have the necessary skills and abilities to perform a job.*
Quantify	*To put something into figures.*
Quartile	*Any three points that divide an ordered distribution into four parts. Each of these parts contain a quarter of the score.*
Quasi-permanent	*Non-permanent method of colouring hair. Fades over a period that is longer than semi-permanent.*
Questionnaire	*A set of questions used for collecting feedback.*
Racist	*Intolerance of race. A person with prejudiced belief that one race is superior (better) than another.*
Radius	*A line running from the centre of the circle to the circumference.*
Rake comb	*Large toothed comb for wet/tangled hair.*
Range	*The difference between the highest and lowest numbers.*
Rapport	*An agreement of trust between hairdresser and client.*
Rash	*Contra-indication response by the body to a chemical.*
Rate of lift	*Lightening of hair colour.*
Ratio	*The comparison of two numbers.*
React	*To respond.*
Reaction	*When chemicals cause a substance to change.*
Rebonding	*Re-fixing amino-acids in the neutralising process to re-form cystine.*
Receding	*Moving from the front to the back gradually.*
Reception	*Greeting.*
Recession areas	*Growth pattern – bald areas around the hairline.*
Recognition	*To identify a thing or person.*
Record card	*Method of recording client's treatments.*
Record	*History of client's treatments.*
Rectify	*To set right.*
Referral	*To suggest or recommend.*
Regenerate	*To renew or replace.*
Regime	*A method or plan.*
Regulate	*Adjust (the temperature of the water).*

Regulations	*Rules.*
Reinforce	*To make information sink in. To confirm.*
Relaxing	*The method of reducing a natural curl by altering the structure either temporarily or permanently using chemicals.*
Relevant information	*The suitability of information based upon your needs.*
Repel	*To reject.*
Represent	*Acting on behalf of someone.*
Reputable	*To have a good reputation.*
Research	*To study something thoroughly.*
Resistant	*To not be affected by.*
Resolution	*The number of pixels per square inch shown on the computer screen. The greater the resolution the better the picture.*
Resolve	*To correct.*
Resources	*Sources of information, expertise and knowledge.*
Respect	*To think of highly.*
Respond	*To answer to.*
Retail	*To be sold.*
Revenue	*Income.*
Review	*To look over and study information again.*
Revision	*To review information in order to remind yourself of its content.*
Ring worm	*A fungal skin infection.*
Rinse	*Process of cleaning, usually with water.*
RIRO	*Rubbish In Rubbish Out (in relation to the Internet).*
Risk assessment	*The process of calculating the risk associated with a hazard and the actions taken to avoid it.*
Risk	*The likelihood of an accident occurring from a hazard.*
Role	*A set of activities or actions attached to a job.*
Roll	*A hairstyle created by folding the hair and securing with pins.*
Roller	*A cylindrical styling tool used to create waves or curls.*
Root lift	*Creating volume at the root.*
Root movement	*Amount of lift achieved at the hair root.*
Root to point	*Winding the hair from the roots to the ends of the hair.*
Rotary massage	*Second massage movement in shampooing using the pads of the fingers in quick, circular movements.*
Round shape	*Face shape suited by flat sides, full on top hair style.*
Rounding off	*Express as a round number (i.e., 4.7 rounded off becomes 5).*
Routine	*A course of action that is followed every day.*
RSI	*Repetitive strain injury. This type of injury occurs from repeated physical movements. It can be caused by bad typing technique, bad posture and lack of adequate rest and breaks. RSI is common in the wrists.*
Sale	*To sell.*
Satisfied	*To be happy with something.*
Scabies	*Raised red lines on the skin caused by itch mite.*
Scalding	*Burning of the skin by a substance (e.g. water) that is too hot.*
Scales	*Outer part of the cuticle.*
Scalp protector	*Product applied to hairline and scalp to protect against chemicals in products.*

Scalp	*Skin of the top of the head.*
Scanning	*To skim/scan text to get a general idea about it.*
Schedule	*To plan a time and place.*
Scissor over comb	*A cutting technique. Scissors are used to cut hair rapidly following the movement over a comb.*
Scrunch drying	*A technique of drying the hair using a diffuser to enhance curls or waves.*
Scum	*Calcium stearate formed from soap and mineral salts in hard water.*
Sea	*Salted water causes damage to hair.*
Search engine	*A program that enables you to locate information on the World Wide Web using keyword searches.*
Sebaceous cyst	*Lump on scalp caused by blocked sebaceous gland.*
Sebaceous gland	*Produces sebum.*
Seborrhoea	*Condition in which excess sebum is produced from the sebaceous gland.*
Sebum	*Oily secretion from the sebaceous gland.*
Secondary colour	*Colours made from mixing primary shades together. Orange, green and violet.*
Section clips	*Used for sectioning hair.*
Section	*Main divisions when dividing the hair for a particular hairdressing service.*
Seminar	*A conference or meeting to discuss a certain subject.*
Semi-permanent colour	*Colour molecules deposited in the hair cuticle or under the open cuticle. They will lighten each time the hair is shampooed.*
Semi-permanent	*Type of colour group (nitro-dyes).*
Sequence	*One thing that follows on to the next.*
Serum	*Product applied during styling to give the hair shine.*
Services	*Alternative name for hair treatment.*
Sesame	*Product used in shampoos for dry scalp.*
Setting comb	*A comb used for finger waving or dressing hair.*
Setting hair	*Setting hair into range of styles and effects.*
Setting mousse	*A product that is applied to wet hair in order to keep style in place.*
Setting pins	*Used for securing rollers in place.*
Shade chart	*Method of identifying the target shade.*
Shadowing	*Following a more experienced member of staff for training purposes.*
Shampoo	*Detergent to wash or clean hair.*
Shine	*Spray lotion applied to hair to achieve a shiny finish.*
Significant figures	*The number of digits expressed in a measurement. Sig. fig. can appear before and/or after the decimal point.*
Signposting guidance	*Within the specifications for the new AS levels, A levels and GNVQs, opportunities for developing or producing evidence for assessment of key skills.*
Simulations	*Activities that simulate or model reality.*
Sincere	*To be genuine.*
Skim-reading	*To skim/scan text to get a general idea about it.*
Skin test	*Application of the product to the skin to assess the reaction.*
Slice colouring technique	*Colouring small sections of hair.*
Slide cutting	*Scissors are slipped through the hair to achieve tapering (feathering) effect.*
Sodium hydroxide	*Lye contained in relaxers.*
Soft water	*Reduced level of mineral content. Water suds easily.*
Software	*A computer program.*

Sparingly	To use a small amount.
Sparse	Not dense. Thin.
Speakers	Device that converts audio signals to sounds that humans can hear.
Specialise	To devote yourself to a particular area of work.
Spell checker	Most computer applications (i.e. Microsoft Word, Excel etc.) will enable you to check documents for incorrect spelling.
Spelling	To form a word with a series of letters.
Spider diagrams	A series of lines and boxes containing relevant information. A form of note taking.
Spiral	Type of setting technique. Also a type of brush that is also known as circular brush.
Spot colouring	Applying colour to certain parts of the hair that need it.
Spreadsheet	A computer program often used to create financial forecasting documents.
Square metre	The area enclosed by a square with sides of one metre long.
Square shape	Shape of face suited by softer hair style and jaw line partially covered.
Stainless steel	A very durable metal.
Stance	The way you stand.
Standard Form	Used so that very large or very small numbers can be written in a more convenient way.
Standards moderation	The means by which awarding bodies ensure consistency across centres and ensure that national standards are being maintained and applied.
State	To express.
Stationery	Paper and office materials.
Statistics	Numerical data.
Sterile	Free from disease causing micro-organisms.
Sterling	Currency of the UK.
Stimulate	To provoke or cause feeling.
Stock	Products held in the salon for sale or treatment.
Stopcock	A valve that opens and closes a gas or water supply pipe.
Straight pins	Strong pins used for long hair styles and holding rollers.
Straighteners	Electrical device used to straighten hair.
Straightening irons	Electrical device used to straighten hair.
Straightening	Method used to make curly hair straight.
Strand test	Test used to monitor colour development.
Strand	Term used for small group of hairs.
Strength	Something that is done well.
Stretch	Test used to measure the tensile strength of hair.
Structure	A build up of parts.
Sturdy	Strong.
Sub divided	To divide something that has already been divided.
Substantive	A thing or idea.
Sulphur	Main chemical of the amino-acid cystine.
Sunlight	Natural light rays that can damage hair.
Supervisor	The person in charge.
Surface conditioner	Work on the surface layer of the hair, coating the hair shaft and filling any gaps in the cuticle layer that have been caused by previous treatments.

Surfactant	Detergent that can damage the hair.
Survey	A method of collecting measured information.
Symmetric	To have equal distribution.
Sympathetically	To be sympathetic. To understand how someone may feel.
Tactful	To show skills in sensing the correct way to deal with others.
Tail comb	Used to help sectioning hair while setting.
Tangled	In a mess.
Tapering	Alternative term for 'feathering'.
Target colour	The hair colour chosen by the client.
Target	Objective set down for staff to reach.
Team working	A group of people working together.
Technician	A person who is trained in the technicalities (small details) of a subject.
Technique	A specific method of working.
Telogen	Stage of hair growth when follicles and papilla are in stage of rest.
Temperature	The heat level.
Temporary	Type of colour group (azo dyes).
Tensile (strength)	Ability of hair to be stretched.
Tension	Stretched.
Terminal	Hair of face, arms, pubic regions.
Test curl	Test to determine if full head can be permed.
Test cut	Test sample of hairs to assess the effect of colouring.
Texture	The coarseness or fineness of hair.
Theme	A subject matter.
Thinning	Reduce the volume of hair.
Timeliness	Reference to the time that information was recorded.
Tinea capitis	Fungal infection, contagious.
Tinting cap	Cap through which strands of hair are pulled to be tinted.
Tinting	Colouring with highlights or lowlights.
Tolerance	The amount that somebody can resist.
Tone	Warm or cool shade of colour tint.
Toner	Colour used to neutralise unwanted tones in lightened hair.
Tool	An implement used for working.
Toxic	Poisonous and harmful.
Tracking	The method by which learner's achievements are recorded across a range of activities.
Traction alopecia	A condition in which the hair falls out due to excessive pulling.
Trainee	A person who is training for a particular job role.
Training	To learn skills.
Transaction	The agreement between a seller and buyer for goods or services.
Transfer	To move from one area to another.
Translucent	Has no colour.
Treatment conditioners	Work by penetrating the cortex and help to repair damage by adding protein. They are known as substantive products.
Treatment	A service.
Trichologist	A specialist in hair and scalp conditions.
Trichorrhexis nodosa	Small white nodules along the hair shaft.

Twist	*A channel of hair that has been wound around itself.*
Twisting	*The method of twisting a channel of hair around itself.*
Ultraviolet	*Type of light ray, can be harmful.*
Unauthorised	*Not allowed.*
Under cut	*To remove hair under the base line.*
Uniform layer cut	*Both sides of the hair cut evenly.*
Uniform	*To be evenly spaced.*
Upper quartile	*Data is split into four equal quarters. The highest quarter is referred to as the upper quartile. For example the upper quartile of 100 is the highest 25 of the numbers.*
Upward nape	*Hair grows upward from the nape.*
UV	*Ultraviolet. Type of light ray, can be harmful.*
VAT	*Value added tax.*
Vellus	*Fine body hair.*
Velocity	*The speed or rate of motion that something is travelling at.*
Vent brush	*Type of brush, creates a broken casual effect.*
Venue	*A place where an event is held.*
Verbal	*Any form of communication that uses words, i.e. speaking and writing in the form of letters, newspapers, emails etc.*
Vigorously	*Active strength.*
Virgin hair	*Hair that has not been chemically treated, bleached.*
Virus	*A tiny organism that causes infectious disease.*
VISA	*Credit card company.*
Vocabulary	*Words and their meanings.*
Volume	*Length x width x height.*
Warm shade	*Colour such as red or orange.*
Warts	*Caused by viral infection of epidermis: non-contagious if not damaged.*
Waste	*To throw away.*
Water soluble	*Dissolves in water.*
Water soluble	*Dissolves in water.*
Water waving	*Another name for finger waving.*
Watermark	*A design that is visible when held up to the light.*
Wax	*A product used during styling and setting, usually made from beeswax.*
Weakness	*Tasks that need improvement in performance.*
Weave cutting	*Scissors 'snip' at roots, creates texture and strengthens root support.*
Weave foil	*Method of tinting hair by placing sections on foil.*
Weaving	*Interlacing hair.*
Web browser	*A software package that allows you to view pages world wide web. Examples are Internet Explorer and Google Chrome.*
Web page	*A document, usually written in HTML (Hypertext Mark-up Language), that can be accessed on the Internet.*
Web Site	*A collection of electronic 'pages'.*
Website	*A collection of electronic 'pages'.*
Weight	*Distribution of hair length within a haircut.*
Wet shampoo	*Shampoo that requires water.*
Whorl	*A growth pattern that follows a circular shape.*

Widows peak	*Growth pattern, hairline points in middle of forehead.*
Winding	*Technique to change the shape of hair.*
Word processor	*A computer program used to create text based documents such as letters and memos, although graphics may also be added.*
World wide web	*The www is a collection of electronic 'pages' that can be accessed over the Internet. The world wide web is NOT the same as the Internet, it is only a part of it.*
Woven hair	*Interlacing hair to other pieces of hair or other items.*
Wrapping lotion	*The product used in the second step of a two-step perm.*
Zinc pyrithione	*Chemical in shampoo that lifts off top layer dead skin cells.*

Index

Numbers in **bold** indicate figures and tables